ACKNOWLEDGEMENTS

This book is dedicated to my wife Dr. Sian Graham whose encouragement was of inestimable value, and to my brother Dr. F. W. Graham whose affliction, early in life, at the hands of the Polio virus, initiated my interest in disorders of the musculo-skeletal system. The book was inspired by the late Dr. Frank Stansfield whose brilliance as an anatomy teacher was well known to many Australian surgeons.

Dr. Scott Harbison's vast experience in orthopaedics and fracture work enabled him to give excellent criticisms and suggestions. I was encouraged also to have the orthopaedic Registrars — always bristling with knowledge — lend their support to this project. Included were Drs. Roger Hargreaves, Paul Stally, David Maxwell, Laurie Kohan and Neville Rowden. The final proof reading was left in the capable hands of Drs. Gary Fettke, Charles New and Ian Barlow.

The line drawings emanated from the skilled hand of the well-known Sydney medical illustrationalist, Julie Eichorn and many of the radiographs were from the extensive collection of Dr. Len Greene. The black and white prints of hand conditions were reproduced with kind permission from the text entitled "A Colour Atlas of Conditions of the Hand" by Bruce Conolly and the Wolfe Publishing Company. The C.T. scans were presented by permission of Dr. S. W. L. Lau and the Medical Journal of Australia and by Drs. Ian Macnab and John McCulloch from their publication "Sciatica and Chymopapain" published by Williams and Wilkins, Baltimore/London, 1983. For the diagrams of ankle injuries I am indebted to Mr. John Crawford Adams and the publishing firm Churchill Livingstone who gave permission for them to be reproduced from "An Outline of Fractures".

Lastly I would like to say that this book would never have experienced a lift off had it not been for the help of Mrs. J. B. Nield.

PREFACE

The questions contained herein, have been derived from the Undergraduate Medical Students Syllabus recommended by the Universities of Sydney and New South Wales.

The purpose of this book is to enable students to test their knowledge by self examination. The assessment may be carried out alone or with the help of someone who may or may not be medically orientated. Considerable value may be obtained if a group of 4 or 5 students utilise the notes with one delivering the questions and the others supplying the answers. The notes are not intended to replace the standard textbooks. A lecturer called upon at short notice, to conduct a teaching session, may use these questions and answers as a basis for his lecture and simply ask these questions of the group thus stimulating interest and encouraging debate.

How to use this book

1. Conceal right side of page.

2. Dwell on each question for 10 seconds unless the answer comes to you instantly.

3. Assess percentage of correct answers.

4. Repeat test in 7 days.

5. Please note, some questions are repeated for emphasis.

6. Questions and answers considered more important for undergraduates are indicated by an asterisk.

Orthopaedics and Fractures

A Question and Answer Study Guide

C. Edmund Graham FRACS, FRCS(Ed), FACS

Butterworths

London   Boston   Singapore   Sydney   Toronto   Wellington

First published 1983 by Standard Publishing House Pty Ltd, Rozelle, NSW
Reprinted 1988 by Butterworths

© **Butterworth & Co. (Publishers) Ltd, 1988**

British Library Cataloguing in Publication Data

Graham, C. Edmund
  Orthopaedics and fractures.
  1. Medicine. Orthopaedics — Questions & Answers
  2. Man. Bones. Fractures
  I. Title
  617′.3′0076

  ISBN 0-407-01188-9

Library of Congress Cataloguing in Publication Data

Graham, C. Edmund.
  Orthopaedics and fractures.

  1. Orthopedia—Examinations, questions, etc.
  2. Fractures—Examinations, questions, etc. I. Title.
  RD732.6.G73 1988   617′.3′0076   88-26233
  ISBN 0-407-01188-9

Printed and bound in England by Page Bros. Ltd, Norwich, Norfolk

Contents

CHAPTER 1

SPINAL INJURIES

Classify cervical spinal injuries into ten groups.

1. Soft tissue sprains and contusion.
2. Wedge compression fracture of vertebral body.
3. Burst fracture of vertebral body.
4. Extension subluxation.
5. Flexion subluxation.
6. Dislocation and fracture dislocation.
7. Fracture of the atlas.
8. Fracture dislocation of atlanto axial joint.
9. Intra spinal displacement of soft tissue.
10. Fracture of spinous process.

It is easy to miss a cervical spinal injury because of the associated ..... injuries.

Head.

How may radiography help to avoid missing an unstable fracture in the cervical spine?

Flexion and extension views should be taken with the lateral radiographs. This will demonstrate any instability that would be missed by a plain lateral in the neutral position.

Why are oblique 45 degree views essential?

These demonstrate the inter-vertebral foramina and the articular processes.

What special radiograph is taken to demonstrate atlas and axis?

A projection through the open mouth is essential for this.

What is the mechanism of the injury to cervical spine?

Excessive movement in any direction can cause these injuries.

A flexion injury alone usually causes what type of fracture?

Wedge compression fracture.

A combined flexion and rotation force usually causes what types of injury? Give three.

Subluxation, dislocation or fracture dislocation.

A flexion or flexion rotation force may also cause a massive displacement of the ..... without bony injury.

Disc.

What might an hyper-extension force produce?

Fracture of the neural arch or dens.

What is the other name for the dens?

Odontoid process.

What might hyper-extension do to the anterior longitudinal ligament and the annulus fibrosus?

These two structures might be ruptured allowing the anterior part of the vertebral bodies to move apart.

What might hyper-extension of an osteo-arthritic cervical spine produce?

Spinal cord impingement by a tough infolded ligamentum flavum.

What fracture may a vertical compression force produce?

A burst fracture of the vertebral body.

What is the difference between a stable and unstable injury to cervical spine?

With a stable injury, the posterior ligaments are intact.

What is the significance of a fracture or injury being stable or unstable?

The stable fracture or injury is not liable to displacement greater than that caused at the time of the injury, whereas an unstable fracture or dislocation is liable to further displacement.

In which injury is external splintage or internal fixation essential?

The unstable injury.

Wedge Compression of Vertebral Body

What force produces wedge compression fracture?

A severe flexion injury may crush the cancellous bone, the compression being most marked in the front of the vertebral body.

Are the posterior ligaments intact?

Yes.

Is the fracture then considered stable or unstable?

Stable.

Is it likely or unlikely with this fracture that the spinal cord will be injured?

Unlikely.

What spinal level is most commonly involved?

12th thoracic or 1st lumbar vertebral body.

Treatment

Would you attempt reduction?

No.

For how long would you support the neck in a collar of plastic or plaster of paris?

Two months.

What advantage does the plastic collar have over plaster of paris?

It can be removed for washing and shaving.

What treatment would you recommend after collar is removed?

Mobilizing and muscle strengthening exercises.

Burst Fracture of Vertebral Body

What force produces a burst fracture?

A vertical compression force transmitted directly along the line of the vertebral bodies while the cervical spine is straight.

What pathological processes take place in a burst fracture? Give two.

The vertebral end plates are ruptured and the inter-vertebral disc is forced into the body of the vertebra.

Bone fragments appear to burst out peripherally in ..... directions.

All.

As a result of the bursting, what might happen to the spinal cord?

Fragments of bone might be driven into it damaging it severely.

Is a burst fracture stable or unstable?

Usually it is stable because the posterior ligaments are intact.

Treatment of Burst Fracture

How would you treat this condition?

Reduction is not necessary and external support is used simply to relieve pain.

How is this provided?

By a polythene collar or plaster of paris collar.

Extension Subluxation

What happens to the anterior longitudinal ligament in this injury?

It is ruptured.

What happens to the vertebral bodies?

The severe extension force separates the bodies anteriorly.

The spine is unstable in ..... .

Extension.

In what positions is the spine stable?

In flexion or in neutral position.

How would you immobilise the neck?

In plaster of paris cast.

For how long?

Eight weeks.

In what position?

Slight flexion.

Flexion Subluxation

In this condition, what happens to the vertebral bodies?

As a result of the injury, one vertebral body is displaced forward upon the other.

What happens to the articular processes?

Nothing — the displacement is not sufficient to cause overriding of these processes.

Occasionally if there is a rotational force as well, there is partial ..... of the articular process on one side.

Overriding.

Does it occur mainly in the upper or the lower half of the cervical spine?

The lower half.

What is the main symptom?

Severe pain with the patient unwilling to move the neck.

How might the displacement be corrected?

Occasionally spontaneously by holding the head erect.

How might this injury be overlooked?

By not having the radiographs taken with the spine flexed and by not taking oblique views.

Are the posterior ligaments damaged?

Yes.

Therefore, if the posterior ligaments are damaged, the condition is regarded as ..... .

Unstable.

Treatment of Flexion Subluxation

What is the first step in management?

Reduce the subluxation.

How is that done?

By extending the cervical spine.

How does one prevent redisplacement?

By holding the neck extended.

How is this extension maintained?

By a plaster collar moulded well down over the sternum.

For how long would you recommend the plaster collar be worn?

Two months.

Does spontaneous fusion ever take place?

Yes, occasionally a buttress of bone forms anteriorly.

What would you recommend if radiographs in flexion and extension show instability persists? — Cervical spinal fusion at the appropriate level would be recommended.

Dislocation and Fracture-dislocation of Cervical Spine

What happens to the articular processes of facet joints in these cases? — They are out of contact and there is overriding of the articular processes.

May the vertebral bodies be compressed? — Yes.

May the neural arch be fractured? — Yes.

Would you consider this fracture unstable? — Yes.

Would you say that transection of the spinal cord is common or rare in this situation? — Common.

Treatment of Dislocation and Fracture-dislocation

Why is careful handling of the patient essential in these cases? — Because of the risk of damage to the spinal cord.

It is best to avoid flexing or extending the .... when moving the patient from the site of the injury. — Entire spine

How is reduction best achieved in dislocation or fracture-dislocation of cervical spine? — By skull traction under X-ray control.

How is the traction applied? — With skull calipers.

How far in do the tips of the calipers go? — Through the outer table of the skull in the parietal region.

How much traction can be applied without giving discomfort yet giving a chance of reducing the dislocation or fracture-dislocation? — Up to 9 kg.

How long may the reduction take after this weight has been applied? — A few hours.

While the traction is being applied, what precautions must be taken? Give two. —
1. Keep a close watch on the neurological state of the upper and lower limbs lest more cord damage is being done.
2. Frequent X-rays to avoid over distraction.

What do you do when the radiographs confirm the articular processes have been disengaged? — Reduction is completed by gradually extending the cervical spine.

How is it held extended? — By maintaining light traction.

After a few days if reduction is considered stable, how would you continue with the immobilization of the neck? — In a plaster of paris or polythene collar.

If there is some doubt as to the degree of stability, what is a better way of treating the patient at this stage? — With traction for three weeks using the skull calipers as mentioned above.

In these unstable fractures then, three weeks' continuous traction in bed is followed by mobilization out of bed wearing a ..... . — Collar.

For how long should the collar be worn at this stage?

For 9-12 weeks.

Indications for Operation for Dislocation and Fracture-dislocation of Cervical Spine

Give two indications.

1. Irreducible locking of articular processes and
2. Persistent instability.

What should you do for irreducible locking of articular processes?

If traction failed, operative reduction with excision of the process if necessary.

This usually happens when reduction with traction has been delayed for ....

A week or so.

What should follow operative excision of the processes?

Fusion of the spine using bone grafts.

With persistent instability, what would you do if gradual redisplacement occurs after an initial reduction and immobilization?

Fusion with the aid of bone grafts at the appropriate levels should be undertaken.

Name two methods of fusing the cervical spine.

Anterior fusion.
Posterior fusion.

With posterior fusion, where is the graft placed?

Between the spinous processes and on the laminae at the same time wiring the spinous processes.

With anterior fusion, where is the bone graft placed?

In a circular bed drilled out by a half inch (1.3 cm) drill between the two adjacent vertebral bodies.

Is surgery becoming more common or less common for cervical dislocations and fracture dislocations?

More common because it lessens the chance of redislocation.

Fracture of the Atlas

How is the atlas fractured?

By a vertical force acting through the skull.

What is the displacement?

The anterior arch and the posterior arch of the atlas are forced open by the impact on occipital condyles.

In which direction do the fragments displace?

Sideways.

Is displacement severe?

No.

Is spinal cord injury common or rare with fracture of the atlas?

Rare.

Cord injury may be evaluated by means of a ..... · ..... scan.

C
T

Treatment

In the absence of injury to the spinal cord, how would you treat this fracture?

Three months in plaster or polythene collar.

Fracture Dislocation of the Atlanto-axial Joint

What two structures give stability to the atlanto-axial joint?

1. Transverse ligament.
2. Anterior arch of the atlas.

What is the other name for the dens?

Odontoid process.

What happens if the dens is fractured?

This permits displacement of the atlas on the axis.

When the dens is fractured at its base, is it displaced together with the atlas or not?

It is displaced together with the atlas usually.

Is the displacement forward or backwards?

It is forward in flexion injuries and backwards in extension injuries.

Which is the more common, forward displacement or backward displacement?

Forward displacement.

Is it possible to have a fracture of the dens without displacement?

Yes.

Why is it difficult to assess the true incidence of this injury?

Because complete severance of the cord at this level is fatal and so the patient rarely reaches the surgeon.

If the patient survives the initial injury, he is likely to be neurologically ..... .

Intact.

How would you treat a fracture dislocation of atlanto-axial joint?

If there is no displacement, place neck in collar of plaster or plastic for 3 months.

If there is displacement, what would you do?

Apply sustained weight traction to skull with calipers, and posture patient to achieve reduction.

For how long would this traction be applied?

Four weeks (because the fracture is unstable).

If local instability should persist, what treatment would you recommend?

Fusion between atlas and axis.

Intra-spinal Displacement of Soft Tissue

In a situation where the radiographs fail to show any bony abnormalities but the patient is tetraplegic or paraplegic, what might be the cause?

Massive disc prolapse or infolding of ligamentum flavum.

With massive disc prolapse, how might you confirm the diagnosis?

With myelography.

Major Fractures and Displacements of the Thoracic and Lumbar Vertebrae

Mechanism of the injury

Fractures of a lumbar or thoracic vertebral body is nearly always caused by a ..... force acting through the long axis of the spinal ..... .

Vertical.
Column.

Give two ways in which this vertical force may be produced.

A fall of weight on to the head as in coal mining or fall onto the feet or buttocks from a height.

Why is the injury to the spine usually a flexion injury?

Because the natural curve of the spine is predominantly one of flexion.

Hyper-flexion injuries are commoner than hyper-extension injuries in the ..... and .....-..... region.

Thoracic and thoraco-lumbar.

What type of fracture might you expect if the compression force is applied when the spinal column is completely straight?

This might produce the burst fracture that has already been described in the cervical region.

In the usual flexion injury then what part of the vertebral body collapses?

The anterior part.

What is the deformity called as a result of this anterior collapse?

Kyphosis.

Is the wedge compression fracture of a vertebral body common or rare?

Common.

What happens if the force is very severe and associated with rotation?

The fracture may be complicated by dislocation of the intervertebral joint with forward displacement of the upper vertebra upon the lower.

What is the main hazard with this type of fracture?

Damage to the spinal cord or cauda equina with associated paralysis.

Wedge Compression Fracture of Vertebral Body

Is it possible for a wedge compression fracture to be overlooked due to the lack of symptoms?

Yes.

Give four symptoms and signs of a compression fracture.

1. Local pain.
2. A prominent spinous process on palpation.
3. Tenderness.
4. Limitation of spinal movements.

In order to avoid missing a compression fracture where there has been a violent injury, what should be done?

Always palpate firmly the length of the spine, that is from the cervical spine to coccyx.

If you have a patient who as a result of a fall has fractured the calcaneus, you should suspect a ..... fracture of the spine.

Compression.

How is this compression fracture finally diagnosed?

With radiographs of thoracic and lumbar spines.

Treatment of Wedge Compression Fracture of Vertebral Body

Is it necessary to reduce the fracture?

No.

Why are these fractures considered stable?

Because the posterior ligaments are intact.

For how long should the patient be hospitalized in bed?

About three weeks.

What physiotherapy would you recommend?

Spinal extension exercises to strengthen the erector spinae muscles.

If the patient complains of severe pain, how might you treat it?

With a plaster or plastic jacket or brace to be worn for three weeks.

Would the plaster be applied with the spine in a neutral position or hyper-extended?

Neutral position.

Would you recommend spinal exercises whilst the plaster is on?

Yes.

Dislocation and Fracture-dislocation of the Thoraco-lumbar Spine

Are these less common or more common than simple wedge compression fractures?

They are less common.

What is the commonest variety of fracture-dislocation in this region?

One in which the fracture-dislocation is such that one vertebra is forced forward upon the vertebra next below.

This injury with one vertebral body slightly forward on the other can take place if one of two things happen with the articular processes. What are they?

1. The articular processes are fractured.
2. The facet joints are dislocated and the two articular processes overridden.

With this injury, what actually happens to the vertebral bodies?

The lower vertebral body is fractured near its upper surface.

Are the posterior ligaments always torn with this injury?

Yes.

Since they are always torn the injury is considered ..... .

Unstable.

If it is considered unstable, what might happen?

Further displacement can easily occur.

These fracture-dislocations take place commonly at what levels? Give two.

1. In the mid thoracic region.
2. At the thoraco-lumbar junction.

What is the commonest type of violence that produces this fracture-dislocation in mid thoracic or thoraco-lumbar junction?

It is always a combined flexion and rotation force.

In what percentage of cases is the spinal cord usually involved?

Almost all of them.

Is the cord injury usually complete?

Yes.

In the lumbar region, however, the injury may only involve the ....

Cauda equina.

Treatment of Dislocation and Fracture-dislocation

What usually overshadows the body injury in these cases?

Paraplegia.

Why must special precautions be taken when transporting these patients who have had a fracture-dislocation?

Because of the risk of causing further damage to an already damaged spinal cord.

If the articular processes are shown to be fractured, how would you proceed with reducing a fracture?

By gently extending the spine with the patient prone.

How would you confirm the reduction?

With radiographs.

Once it is seen to be reduced, for how long would you immobilize the spine?

Three months.

How is this achieved?

With a plaster or polythene jacket.

In what position is the patient while this plaster is being applied?

Prone and with spine slightly extended.

If the articular processes are overridden but not fractured, why would you be reluctant to attempt closed reduction?

Because it is unlikely to succeed and forced extension might further damage the spinal cord or cauda equina.

How, therefore, would you proceed in this case where the facet/articular processes are overridden but not fractured?

At open operation, reduction is obtained under direct vision.

How is the reduction held once it has been achieved? Give three.

1. By a plate and screws.
2. Wire fixed to the spinous processes.
3. Harrington or other rods.

Would you immobilize it in a plaster jacket after this operation?

Yes, for three months.

Minor Fractures of the Spinal Column

How would you treat a fracture of the transverse process in the lumbar region?

Rest in bed until the acute pain subsides.
After that, give heat and exercises.
After two or three weeks, the patient is up and about.

Fracture of the Sacrum

How is this produced?
Give two.

1. A fall on the sacrum.
2. A direct blow to the sacrum.

Is this fracture usually a crack or a widely displaced injury?

Usually a crack.

How is it treated?
Give two.

Bed rest and analgesics until the pain passes off.

Fracture of the Coccyx

How is this produced?

By a fall on the "tail".

How is it treated?

Bed rest and analgesics till pain subsides.

If pain persists and is very uncomfortable, what might be recommended?

Excision of coccyx.

Burst Fracture of Vertebral Body

How is this produced?

The vertical compression force is applied with the spine straight in these cases, whereas with the wedge compression, the spine is slightly flexed during the moment of impact.

With the burst fracture, what happens to the intervertebral disc?

It is forced into the affected vertebral body.

With the burst fracture, in which direction do the spicules of bone travel?

In all directions.

In which direction might posterior fragments be directed?

Into the spinal cord or cauda equina.

Which of these fractures then, the wedge compression fracture or the burst fracture, is the more serious?

The burst fracture because of the risk to the spinal cord or cauda equina.

With a burst fracture, are the posterior ligaments intact?

Yes, so therefore the spine is considered stable.

Treatment of burst fracture.

The same as for compression fracture, that is, wear a surgical corset for three weeks, after initial period of bed-rest.

The Nerve Injury in Paraplegia from Spinal Injuries

At the thoraco-lumbar junction, the lower segment of the spinal cord and the proximal ..... of the .... lie side by side in the spinal canal.

Roots.
Cauda equina.

What significance does the presence of these two structures have with thoraco-lumbar fracture-dislocation?

The lesion might be a mixed one due partly to cord injury and partly to nerve root injury.

If the lesion is incomplete, what nearly always suffers?

The cord suffers and the nerve roots usually escape injury.

What is the expression used for this phenomenon?

It is called lumbar root escape.

Below the first lumbar vertebrae, what part of the spinal cord do we have?

There is no spinal cord but the cauda equina.

Is the cauda equina more resistant to injury than the cord itself?

Yes. So the injury may, therefore, be incomplete.

Characteristics of Complete Transection of the Cord

What is the immediate consequence of division of the cord?

Total suppression of function in segments below the lesion.

What is the other name for total suppression of function in the segments below the lesion?

Spinal shock.

The initial paralysis is flaccid or spastic. Which?

Flaccid.

Is the sensory loss complete?

Yes.

Are the visceral reflexes exaggerated or suppressed?

Suppressed.

How long does spinal shock last?

Usually a few days or sometimes weeks.

As the spinal shock passes off, what happens to the paralysis?

It becomes spastic instead of flaccid.

How does this manifest itself?

The reflexes, both visceral and tendon, become exaggerated.

What else happens to reflexes?

They are unmodified by higher control.

If reflex activity returns without recovery of sensibility or voluntary power, what do you conclude?

This is diagnostic of complete transection of the spinal cord.

Why is it not possible to make an unequivocal diagnosis of complete transection of the cord 48 hours after the injury?

Because of the temporary phenomena of spinal shock.

Give two signs that indicate incomplete transection of the cord.

1. Early return of voluntary motor power.
2. Sensory perception below the level of the lesion.

Characteristics of Severe Injury of the Cauda Equina

Is the paralysis flaccid or spastic with cauda equina lesions?

Flaccid throughgout.

What happens to the tendon and visceral reflexes with severe injury to the cauda equina?

These are abolished and do not return unless nerve fibres recover their pre-injury function.

The Bladder

Whereabouts is the reflex centre which governs normal emptying of the bladder?

In the second and third sacral segments of the spine.

Whence does the overriding control emanate?

From the cerebral cortex.

What happens then with transection of the cord above the sacral segments?

The overriding cerebral control is cut off.

What happens to the sacral reflex centres in 2nd and 3rd segments?

They are left intact.

What happens in the early weeks after injury in these cases where the overriding control of the cerebral cortex is cut off?

There is firstly retention of urine with overflow.

What happens after an interval of a few weeks or a few months?

The reflex centres in the cord take over and control automatic emptying of the bladder when it is filled to a certain capacity.

What is this reflex state called?

The automatic bladder or cord bladder.

What happens if the nerve pathways or reflex control of the bladder are severed in a sacral segment injury?

True reflex emptying does not occur and the patient is left with periodic emptying of the bladder.

Upon what does this autonomic bladder depend?

Local reflexes in the bladder wall give rise to periodic emptying.

How may emptying of the autonomic bladder be completed?

By pressing on the abdomen or by abdominal straining.

How then does an automatic bladder differ from an autonomic bladder?

The automatic bladder depends on the spinal cord and the sacral reflex being intact whereas the autonomic bladder depends upon the reflex in the muscle of the bladder wall itself.

Special Dangers in Cases of Spinal Paraplegia

Name two areas of infection that might be fatal in the first few months after developing spinal paraplegia.

1. Urinary tract infection.
2. Infection of pressure sores.

Prognosis: is it possible for the spinal cord to recover after complete transection?

No.

Is there any chance of recovery in the roots of the cauda equina?

Yes, because they behave like peripheral nerves in their capacity for recovery.

Under what conditions are these so-called peripheral nerves able to recover?

If their sheaths remain patent and in continuity.

Since the spinal nerve roots are similar to peripheral nerves, what might you expect with neuro-praxia?

Recovery may occur early.

A nerve that has undergone axonotmesis may do what?

Regenerate.

Neurotmesis in the region is ..... .

Irrecoverable.

One would conclude then that cauda equina injuries are more favourable than ..... injuries.

Cord.

Treatment of Paraplegia

Where is the best place to treat these patients?

In a special spinal unit.

Management of the Fracture

If in the cervical region a severe fracture dislocation is seen, how would you proceed?

Reduce the fracture-dislocation with skull calipers and proceed as mentioned above.

If there be no body displacement but severe paralysis, how would you proceed?

Perform myelography to see if the paralysis is due to a protruded inter-vertebral disc and then if it is, operate and remove it to decompress the cord.

With regard to fracture-dislocation of the thoracic spine, why is open operation, reduction and fixation with plate and screws recommended?

Because there is always doubt as to how much chance there is of recovery taking place and it is felt that the patient has a better chance if all pressure is taken off the cord, and because the treatment of the paraplegic in plaster is fraught with complications.

With regard to thoraco-lumbar junction fractures or lumbar fractures in these two areas, why is surgery indicated immediately?

Neurological injury is more likely to be incomplete, at least some of the nerve roots being spared.

What are the purposes of operation on the lumbar region?

1. One may reduce any gross displacement under direct vision to ensure the roots of the cauda equina are free from pressure.
2. To provide internal fixation to prevent re-displacement.
3. To simplify nursing.

Nursing

Is there ever an indication to nurse the patient in plaster jacket or plaster bed?

No.

Upon what should the patient be placed?

Soft pillows.

How often should the patient be turned?

Every two hours throughout day and night.

How many sides of the patient should be utilized for this therapy?

All four sides, front, back, left side and right side.

Care and Training of the Bladder

In the management of the bladder, why was suprapubic cystostomy abandoned. Give two reasons.

1. It failed to prevent infection.
2. It led to bladder shrinkage.

What is the modern method for controlling bladder function? Give two.

1. Intermittent catheterization.
2. Many surgeons prefer an indwelling catheter.

What precautions must be taken with catheterization?

The asepsis must be very strict.

How is infection prevented? Give two methods.

1. By using antibiotics.
2. By strict aseptic technique when the catheter is changed.

How is periodic emptying of the bladder achieved?

By allowing the bladder to fill almost to capacity between catheterizations and then by draining at regular intervals usually four times a day.

With regard to the automatic bladder, how long does it take for emptying to become established?

Within one to three months.

In cases where the sacral segments are destroyed, we are left with an ..... bladder.

Autonomic.

How satisfactory is this type of bladder?

Not highly satisfactory.

How does one help this bladder emptying?

By abdominal straining or manual compression.

Name three features of rehabilitation.

1. Maintenance of morale in spite of the difficulty of the problems.
2. Re-education to do a job.
3. Encouragement toward competitive sports all help.

CHAPTER 2

FRACTURES OF THE NECK AND SHAFT OF THE HUMERUS AND OF THE SHOULDER GIRDLE

Fractures of the Humerus

* Classify fractures of the humerus into six groups.

1. Fracture of the neck of the humerus.
2. Fracture of the greater tuberosity.
3. Fracture of the shaft of humerus.
4. Supra condylar fracture.
5. Fractures of the condyles.
6. Fractures of the epicondyle.

Fractures of the Neck of the Humerus

* Are these fractures common in younger or older people?

Older people and to a lesser extent in teenagers.

* Is it commoner in men or women?

Women.

* How is the fracture produced?

By a fall on the outstretched hand.

* Give two types of displacement.

1. There may be no displacement.
2. There may be moderate or severe tilting of the head segment due to the shaft being either abducted or adducted.

* In what proportion of cases are fractures of the neck of humerus impacted?

Over 50%.

* What is the significance of the fracture being impacted?

It doesn't need internal fixation or any special immobilizing force other than a sling.

Diagnosis

* This is usually made out by the history and type of injury.
  Give one indication that might make you feel the fracture is impacted.

The limb may be moved passively through a reasonable range without causing severe pain if the fracture is impacted.

Treatment

* With regard to treatment, is the following statement true or false?
  In most cases, the most satisfactory method of treatment is one which permits early mobilization of the shoulder even if an imperfect position of the fracture is accepted.

True.

Give two methods whereby the greater tuberosity may be fractured.

1. A fall on the abducted arm brings tuberosity into heavy contact with the acromion process.
2. Rarely, the supraspinatus may avulse the tuberosity.

Unimpacted Fractures

* How long would you immobilize these?

In a sling (plus or minus a bandage to hold arm to chest) for three weeks.

* What treatment would you suggest after that?

Active mobilizing exercises.

In younger patients with unimpacted fracture, how might you immobilize them?

In an abduction splint or a shoulder spica for 4 weeks after the fracture has been manipulated into the correct position.

If operative reduction is necessary for a fracture of the neck of the humerus, how would you hold it? Give two.

1. Intramedullary nail.
2. Metal plate fixed with screws.

Give two complications of fractures of neck of humerus.

1. Stiffness is very common in the older age group.
2. Nerve injury.

What nerve may be injured? Give two effects of this injury.

Circumflex nerve.
1. Deltoid muscle weakness with restriction of abduction of the shoulder.
2. Numbness over outer side of upper arm area.

One further complication of this fracture is dislocation of the shoulder. How would you manage this fracture-dislocation?

The fracture should be treated along the usual lines after the dislocation has been reduced.

Fractures of the Shaft of the Humerus

* What is the commonest location of a humeral shaft fracture?

Middle third.

* Name two forces that can produce these fractures.

1. Indirect twisting force giving a spiral fracture.
2. Direct force giving a transverse fracture.

Is there a particular age group?

No.

Is it uncommon in children?

Yes.

With what disease are fractures of the proximal half of the humerus commonly associated?

Pathological fracture due to carcinomatous metastases.

Treatment

* Is it necessary to secure perfect end to end apposition?

No.

* Is it necessary to enforce strict immobilization?

No.

* Following reduction, two types of plaster might be used to hold the fracture. What are they?

A hanging cast known as a U slab extends from axilla to the outer deltoid region via the olecranon.
Occasionally a complete cast including the forearm is used with the elbow at right angles.

* Further immobilization with these two casts is provided by a ..... and ....

Collar and cuff.

* When the fragments are unstable, how might immobilization be achieved?

A plaster shoulder spica to include the trunk and the whole upper limb may be effective.

* If this cumbersome plaster shoulder spica is to be avoided, name two ways in which internal fixation might be used to achieve the same end.

1. Plate and screws.
2. Intramedullary nail.

Name one important complication of intramedullary nailing.

Inhibition of shoulder movement due to protrusion of the nail above the greater tuberosity.

How might this be obviated?

By inserting the nail (preferably closed) from below upward, the nail being made to enter from just above the olecranon fossa.

Complications of Fracture of the Shaft of the Humerus

* Which nerve might be injured?

Radial nerve.

* Why is this one nerve likely to be injured?

Because it comes in contact with bone in the spiral groove.

* Is the injury usually a contusion or a complete division?

Usually a contusion.

* What motor changes would you expect with a radial nerve palsy?

Wrist drop.

* Name 5 muscle groups that are paralysed when the radial nerve is injured.

Extensors of the wrist.
Extensors of the fingers.
Extensors of the thumb.
Brachio radialis muscle.
Supinator muscle.

* What sensory loss might be noted?

A small area of anaesthesia is noted on the radial side of the back of the hand.

Treatment of Radial Nerve Palsy

In the first instance it is assumed that the nerve is in continuity and spontaneous ..... is awaited.

Recovery.

Whilst awaiting recovery, how would you manage the patient? Give two.

1. Exercises to wrist and fingers.
2. Cock up (or dorsiflexing) splint will prevent contractures.

If after six weeks the nerve function is still absent, what would you recommend?

Exploration of the nerve, with a view to restoring continuity with the aid of micro surgery.

If nerve function is permanently absent, what procedures might be undertaken to restore dorsi flexion of the wrist?

Tendon transfer operations.

Name four tendon transfers that might be used to restore dorsi flexion to the wrist in case of radial palsy of a permanent nature.

Pronator teres transfer to extensor carpi radialis brevis. Flexor carpi ulnaris or flexor carpi radialis transfer to extensor digitorum and extensor pollicis longus.
Palmaris longus is transferred to abductor pollicis longus.

Name one further complication of fractures of the humeral shaft.

Non-union.

Give two ways of treating non union of a fractured humeral shaft.

Plate and screws and bone graft or intramedullary nail and bone graft.

Whence is the bone graft derived?

Usually iliac crest or occasionally from a slab of tibia.

Give three less common complications of fracture of the humerus.

1. Delayed union.
2. Non union.
3. Stiff shoulder.

Fractures of the Shoulder Girdle

Name two bones that are to be discussed with fractures of the shoulder girdle.

1. Fractures of the clavicle.
2. Fractures of the scapula.

Fractures of the Clavicle

* Are fractures of the clavicle due to a direct blow or a fall on the outstretched hand?

Fall on the outstretched hand.

* Are fractures of the clavicle common or rare?

Common.

* Which is the commoner site for fractures of the clavicle — in the inner or outer third?

At the junction of the middle and outer thirds.

* When fractures occur in the outer third, the outer fragment of bone is pulled ..... and it is also displaced ..... .

Downwards.
Medially.

* So fractures of the clavicle and scapula are grouped together as fractures of the ..... girdle.

Shoulder.

* A fall on the outstretched hand is the commonest method of sustaining a fracture of the ..... and the commonest site for a fracture of the clavicle is at the junction of the ..... and ..... thirds.

Clavicle.

Middle; Outer.

* The displacement of the bones with a fractured clavicle is simply that the lateral fragment is displaced in two directions. What are they?

Downwards and Medially — due to weight of the arm.

Treatment of Fractures of the Clavicle

* The classical treatment is with a firm ..... of ..... bandage.

Figure.
Eight.

* This has the effect of pulling the shoulders backward and overcoming the ..... and ..... displacement of the outer fragment.

Downwards; Medial.

* Should the figure of eight bandage be applied too tightly, the ..... return from the upper limb may be obstructed.

Venous.

* A figure of eight bandage too tightly applied might damage what other structures in the axilla?

One or more nerve trunks.

* Is it essential to get precise end to end togetherness of a fractured clavicle? — No, because union usually takes place satisfactorily with imperfect positioning.

* In addition to the figure of eight bandage, a ..... is used. — Sling.

* How long after sling and figure of eight immobilization would one start exercising the shoulder joint? — Seven days.

* How long is the figure of eight bandage retained? — Two weeks.

* The commonest residual disability with a fracture of a clavicle is a ..... at the fracture site. — Lump.

* In children, remodelling quickly restores a normal ..... . — Contour.

* In adults, however, irregularities and lump formation might remain and if these are a nuisance, then they can be removed ..... . — Surgically.

* In older patients, if the shoulder joint is not exercised early on, then ..... might be a nuisance. — Stiffness.

Fractures of the Scapula

Are fractures of the scapula common or rare? — Rare.

Name four fractures of the scapula. —
1. Fracture of the body of scapula.
2. Fracture of the neck of scapula.
3. Fracture of the acromion process.
4. Fracture of the coracoid process.

Fractures of the Body of the Scapula

These fractures are splinted by the scapula's own ..... attachments. — Muscle.

Splinting, therefore, is not needed for this rare fracture and a simple ..... immobilization is instituted until the pain passes off. — Sling.

..... exercises are begun as soon as pain has disappeared. — Shoulder.

Likewise, with fractures of the neck of the scapula, the fracture line does not usually involve the ..... and the fracture line normally runs from the ..... notch to the ..... border. — Glenoid
Scapula; Axillary.

Treatment of the fractures of the neck of the scapula usually requires sling immobilization alone until the ..... passes off and then ..... are instituted. — Pain; Exercises.

The glenoid fragment in fractures of the neck of the scapula may be displaced ..... . — Downwards.

Fractures of the Acromion Process

There are two fractures that involve the acromion process. One might be a simple ..... without displacement and the other fracture of the acromion process might be a comminuted one with the displacement that is ..... .

Crack.

Downwards.

Treatment of Fractures of the Acromion

If the fracture is simply a crack with minimal displacement, a sling is worn for a week or so and then active ..... are commenced.

Exercises.

If the acromion is comminuted or markedly depressed, it is more satisfactory to ..... the acromion back to the ..... joint.

Excise.
Acromio-clavicular.

In this event, what would you do with the deltoid muscle that is attached to the acromion?

Resuture the deltoid muscle to stump of acromion.

The deltoid muscle following this operation is then relaxed by holding the arm at 90 degrees in an ..... frame for a .... period.

Abduction; Three week.

Fractures of the Coracoid Process

Fractures of the coracoid process might be a simple ..... or if it is a complete fracture, the displacement is such that the tip of the process is displaced ..... .

Crack.

Downwards.

What muscles do you think pull the coracoid downwards?

The coraco-brachialis and the biceps (short head).

No matter which one of these two fractures is sustained, the treatment is simply disregard the ..... and commence ..... as soon as possible.

Fracture; Exercises.

CHAPTER 3

SHOULDER DISLOCATION AND FRACTURES OF THE SHAFT OF THE HUMERUS

* There are two main types of shoulder dislocation and they are ..... and ..... .

Anterior; Posterior.

* By far the commoner type of dislocation is the ..... one.

Anterior.

* The anterior dislocation is produced by a force that pushes the head of the humerus in an anterior direction. The head of the humerus can be displaced forward when one falls on to the outstretched hand. Before the head of the bone can go forward, however, it must tear or detach the ..... of the joint.

Capsule.

* Occasionally a part of the head of the bone is ..... as it moves forwards over the rim of the glenoid.

Crushed.

* From our knowledge of anatomy, one can calculate three types of anterior dislocation that one is likely to meet. The head of the bone can slip below the glenoid and this is then called a ....

Sub glenoid dislocation.

* The next one is that the head may move forwards and be lodged under the coracoid process. This is then known as a ....

Sub coracoid dislocation.

* The head may also move to occupy a position under the clavicle and this is then known as a ....

Sub clavicular dislocation.

Acute Dislocation of the Shoulder

Is shoulder dislocation more common in adults or adolescents?

Adults.

How is a posterior shoulder dislocation produced? Give three methods.

1. By a direct blow to the front of the shoulder driving the humeral head backwards.
2. Electric shock.
3. Epileptic fit.

* **Clinical features of anterior dislocation:**
* Name the two common symptoms.

1. Very severe pain.
2. Inability to move the shoulder joint.

* On physical examination, the outstanding sign is that of loss of ..... of the shoulder below the tip of the acromion.

Contour.

The rigid abducted arm appears ....

Too long.

* As a result, the most lateral point of the shoulder region becomes the ..... process.

Acromion.

* How is the dislocation confirmed?

By radiographs that show the humeral head displaced out of the glenoid fossa.

With regard to posterior dislocation, what is the most obvious sign?

Fixed medial rotation of the arm.

Attempts to externally rotate the arm are met with ..... .

Resistance.

Does an antero-posterior radiograph show the posterior dislocation clearly?

Not always. A lateral projection is more accurate.

Why is a radiograph essential?

To exclude a coexisting fracture.

Treatment of Acute Dislocation of the Shoulder

* How is the pain of reduction alleviated?

By general anaesthesia.

* Give two methods whereby anterior dislocation may be reduced.

1. The Kocher method.
2. The Hippocratic method.

* Give the four steps in the Kocher method.

1. With the elbow flexed to a right angle, steady traction is applied in the line of the humerus.
2. The arm is rotated laterally.
3. The arm is adducted by passing the elbow across the body toward the mid line.
4. The arm is rotated medially so that the hand falls across the opposite side of the chest.

* How is the Hippocratic method performed?

Place the stockinged foot of the surgeon into the axilla and apply a steady pull on the semi-abducted arm in the long axis of the humerus. The stockinged foot levers the head of the humerus from under the glenoid rim and the muscles then pull the head back into the glenoid.

After reduction, for how long is sling immobi-zation instituted?

About three weeks.

How does one reduce a posterior dislocation of shoulder joint?

Under general anaesthesia, rotate the arm laterally while a direct force is applied to the back of the humeral head.

* **Complications of acute dislocation of shoulder joint:**
* Give four complications.

1. Injury to circumflex nerves.
2. Injury to brachial plexus.
3. Injury to axillary artery.
4. Associated fracture of greater tuberosity of the humerus and occasionally fracture of the neck of the humerus.

* What is the consequence of circumflex nerve injury?

Paralysis of deltoid muscle plus anaesthesia of the lateral aspect of the upper arm.

* How would you treat this nerve injury?

In most cases, the treatment is expectant and recovery takes place in a few weeks or months.

Recurrent Anterior Dislocation of the Shoulder

* If the capsule is stripped from the anterior margin of the glenoid rim, the head of the humerus readily dislocates under what circumstances?

When the arm is abducted and extended and rotated laterally.

* This defect in the capsular attachment enables recurrent dislocation to take place with considerable inconvenience to the patient.

Treatment of Recurrent Dislocation of the Shoulder Joint

Is an operation essential?

Yes.

Name three operations to cure recurrent dislocation of the shoulder.

1. Bankart.
2. Putti Platt.
3. Bristow's Operation.

* In essence, the Bankart operation implies reattachment of the .... to the glenoid.

Capsular labrum.

* The re-attachment is best performed with the aid of ....

Wire sutures.

* The Putti Platt operation is one in which the capsule of the joint in front and the sub-scapularis muscle are .... in like fashion to a double breasted coat.

Over lapped.

What is Bristow's Operation?

The detached coracoid process is screwed to a raw area in front of the neck of scapular thus creating a bony block to anterior dislocation.

* With regard to shoulder dislocations generally, it is safe to assume that if the shoulder or if the head of the humerus can be dislocated forward, it could also be dislocated ..... .

Backwards.

* The backward dislocation is known as the ....

Posterior dislocation of the shoulder joint.

* This type of dislocation is extremely ..... .

Rare.

Fractures of the Shaft of the Humerus

* **Causes of fractures of the shaft of the humerus:**
* A twisting force causes a ..... fracture.

Spiral.

* A direct blow on the humerus causes a ..... fracture.

Transverse.

* **Physical signs:**
* On inspecting the limb, one can frequently see ..... .

Deformity.

* On palpating the limb, ... is a feature.

Tenderness.

* Attempts at moving the limb gives rise to .....

Pain.

* When considering movements it is most important that the fingers be moved to make quite sure there is no ..... injury.

Nerve.

* A fracture of the humerus is most likely to involve the ..... nerve.

Radial.

* Why do you think the radial nerve is the one most likely to be involved?

Because it is in contact with the bone in its mid section.

* The final investigation of course, is the ..... .

Radiograph.
The radiograph shows a fracture whether it be of the spiral or transverse type.

Treatment of Fractures of the Shaft of the Humerus

* As is the usual way, we consider this under four headings — name them:
  ....
  ....

1. Reduce   2. Hold reduced
3. How long   4. Soft parts.

* Whose name do you associate with this method of approach to a fracture?

Graham Apley of St. Thomas's Hospital, London.

* In considering the reduction, this is usually carried out simply by ..... .

Gravity.

* When considering holding the fracture reduced, the technique is to allow the weight of the arm to pull the humerus straight. This is achieved in a U-shaped plaster that extends from the acromion process down under the olecranon and up again to the ..... .

Axilla.

* This U-shaped plaster is bound on by a crepe bandage and exerts traction by virtue of its weight. In addition to the U-shaped plaster which is pulling downward towards the floor, the forearm has to be supported with the aid of a ..... .

Sling.

* These fractures usually take six weeks to unite if they are of the ..... or ..... type.

Spiral; Comminuted.

* If these fractures are of the transverse type, then obviously the duration of immobilization will be ..... .

Longer.

* In actual practice, the transverse fracture usually takes ..... weeks to become firm.

Six.

* With regard to the soft parts, it is important that exercises are carried out to the ..... , ... and ..... joints.

Wrist; Fingers
Shoulder.

31

CHAPTER 4

BRACHIAL PLEXUS INJURIES

Brachial plexus injuries are a major cause of partial or complete loss of function in which limb?

The upper limb.

In which direction is the violent force on shoulder or upper limb usually applied in cases of brachial plexus injuries?

Downward away from the neck.

A heavy downward blow on the shoulder, for example, would damage the upper or lower roots of the brachial plexus. Which?

The upper roots, i.e. C5, C6 and C7.

When a motor cyclist comes off his machine and his shoulder hits a telegraph post while he is travelling horizontally, what might happen to the upper roots of the brachial plexus. Give three.

1. The roots may be stretched.
2. The roots may be torn.
3. The roots may be avulsed from the spinal cord.

What three upper limb movements are lost as a result of this lesion to the upper roots of the brachial plexus?

1. Loss of abduction of the shoulder.
2. Loss of lateral rotation of the shoulder.
3. Loss of flexors of the elbow.

* The limb then is left in the ..... tip position.

Porter's.

* This type of paralysis is known as the ..... type of paralysis.

Erb.

* How is the other type of brachial plexus injury sustained, i.e. the Klumpke type?

By forcible elevation of the arm and shoulder as in a difficult breech delivery.

* Which roots would you expect this to stretch?

The lower roots, i.e. C8 and T1.

* Where is the motor and sensory loss in this type of lesion usually?

In the forearm and hand.

* What type of paralysis is this called?

Klumpke.

* In the more severe injuries, the whole plexus is torn or avulsed and this leaves a totally ..... arm.

Paralysed.

Brachial Plexus Lesions in Infants

* These injuries are commonly caused during delivery of the baby.
  Which type of delivery is most likely to cause brachial plexus injuries?

Breech delivery.

* During the breech delivery the shoulder is pulled away from the head so what type of lesion would you expect?

The upper arm type or Erb.

* Soon after birth it is noticed that the child doesn't move the arm normally. Give two other conditions that can cause failure of the normal use of the arm after childbirth.

1. Fractures of the upper limb.
2. Hemiplegia.

* With Erb's Palsy, the arm is held in the Porter's Tip position. What is that position?

The arm is adducted to the side and medially rotated.

* If the arm is left in that position, what might develop?

Secondary contractures.

* Do most cases recover or is paralysis usually permanent?

Most cases recover although it may take many months.

* If the lower roots of the brachial plexus are involved in a birth injury, what is the condition called?

Klumpke type of paralysis.

* Which is the commoner, Erb's or Klumpke?

Erb's paralysis.

Treatment of Brachial Plexus Lesions in Infants

* How does the mother prevent fixed contractures developing?

By moving the limb frequently through a full range.

* Where permanent paralysis has set in, name three possible operations that might be performed to improve function of the limb.

1. Corrective osteotomy.
2. Arthrodesis of the shoulder.
3. Tendon transfer operation.

Brachial Plexus Lesions in Adults

* Brachial plexus injuries are usually caused in adults by what type of accident?

Motor cycle crashes.

* How does one ascertain which nerve has been involved?

By physical examination testing motor and sensory phenomena etc.

* How would you diagnose an avulsion of the roots of the plexus from the spinal cord?

By myelography.

Treatment of Brachial Plexus Lesions in Adults

* With avulsed roots the outlook is very poor and there are just two procedures which must be considered. What are they?

Amputation of the useless limb, through the mid-humerus plus shoulder arthrodesis. Some reconstructive operation might be contemplated.

* If the roots of the plexus are not avulsed, what operation may be carried out?

Exploration of brachial plexus and suturing of injured nerves might be worthwhile, using grafts and microsurgical techniques.

* Does surgery carry a good or poor prognosis?

Usually poor.

With incomplete lesions, how long may recovery take?

2–3 years.

CHAPTER 5

SUPRACONDYLAR FRACTURE OF THE HUMERUS

* This fracture is much commoner in ...... than in ....

Childhood.
Adulthood.

* Is it common or rare?

Very common.

* Why is the fracture of great importance?

Because of the risk of injury to the brachial artery.

* How is the fracture sustained?

By a fall on the outstretched hand with the elbow bent.

* When there is displacement, the lower fragment is displaced and tilted ..... and twisted ....
Give two clinical features.

Backwards.
Inwards.
Pain and deformity.

Treatment of Supracondylar Fracture of the Humerus

* If there is no displacement of the fragment, the child's limb is simply placed in a plaster or a sling for ..... weeks.

Three.

* If the fracture is displaced with the lower fragment tilted backwards and displaced backwards, then ..... reduction under .... should be undertaken.

Manipulative; General Anaesthesia

* To reduce this fracture, the lower fragment obviously having been displaced and angulated backwards has to be pushed ..... with direct pressure behind the olecranon after applying a longitudinal traction on the limb.

Forward.

..... or ..... displacement of lower fragment may also require correction.

Medial; lateral.

* The elbow is then flexed to about ..... degrees.

Ninety.

How does one confirm accurate reduction?

With radiographs in two planes.

* After reduction, the limb is immobilized in a .... with the elbow flexed a little more acutely than ....

Plaster of paris slab or collar and cuff.
Ninety degrees.

* If elbow flexion causes Radial Pulse obliteration, how may you proceed?

Apply Dunlop traction with arm abducted and elbow straight — maintain for three weeks.

* Perfect anatomical reposition is not essential, but ..... tilting of the ..... fragment should be corrected.

Lateral; Lower.

Percutaneous .... may hold the fracture if persistently unstable.

Kirschner wires.

* The flexing of the elbow is important for the maintenance of the lower fragment in its corrected .... .

Position.

* A careful watch has to be kept on the ..... in the forearm and hand, therefore, the child is kept in hospital for 24 hours after the reduction and the Sister in charge of the ward instructed regarding the regular half-hourly observation on the ..... pulse.

Circulation.

Radial.

* The plaster of paris supporting the limb should be cut away at the site of palpation of the radial ..... .

Pulse.

How long does union take?

Three weeks.

* The three main complications of this fracture are:

1. Injury to the brachial artery.
2. Injury to the median nerve.
3. Malunion with consequent deformities.

Arterial Occlusion

* If left untreated, arterial occlusion gives rise to what condition?

Volkmann's Ischaemic Contracture.

* The brachial artery may be occluded from without or from within, or by virtue of spasm in the ..... of the artery.

Wall.

* What might occlude the artery from without? Give three factors.

1. Bone fragment.
2. Blood and oedema.
3. A tight plaster cast.

* What might occlude the artery from within? Give one.

Thrombosis.

* What might cause narrowing of the arterial lumen from within the wall of the artery?

Spasm of the vessel wall.

* Arterial occlusion in most cases produces ischaemic changes in the muscles of the ..... and sometimes in the peripheral ..... .

Forearm.
Nerves.

* Since the blood supply has been reduced, the affected muscles in the front of the forearm are replaced by ..... tissue.

Fibrous.

* What normally happens to fibrous tissue?

It contracts and draws the wrist and fingers into flexion.

* What is the name of this flexion deformity?

Volkmann's Ischaemic Contracture.

* Injury to the peripheral nerve trunks gives rise to malfunction of the nerves. What are the two components?

Sensory and motor components.

* As a result of this, there may be permanent weakness and sensory loss in the front of the forearm and hand.

For how long can a major peripheral nerve withstand total ischaemia before damage becomes apparent?

2—4 hours.

What about muscle ischaemia?

After 6—8 hours it never recovers.

* In the diagnosis of arterial occlusion in addition to diminution or absence of the radial pulse, one sees that the fingers are ....., ... and ..... and in addition, pain can be produced by passively ..... the fingers.

Cold,
Pink; Numb.
Extending.

In summary, what are the six P's of Volkmann's Ischaemia?

The limb is:
1. Painful
2. Pale (or)
3. Plum coloured
4. Pulseless
5. Paraesthetic
6. Paralysed.

* Marked pain in the forearm then is observed if the fingers are passively ..... .

Extended.

* Once Volkmann's Ischaemic Contracture is established, of course, the condition is diagnosed by the characteristic .... of wrist and fingers.

Flexion contracture.

Treatment of Arterial Occlusion in Supracondylar Fractures

* In the early stages, the occlusion of the artery must be considered an emergency, because the effects are ..... after a few hours.

Irreversible.

* What is the first thing to do?

Remove the external splint and straighten the elbow.

* In addition, hot bottles are applied over the other three ..... in order to promote general ..... .

Limbs
Vaso-dilatation.

Keep the limb ..... to reduce metabolic needs.

Cool.

* If after ..... minutes the circulation is still impaired, then the brachial artery has to be ..... .

Thirty.

Explored.

* At surgery, any ..... or .... pressing on the artery must be removed.

Bone; Soft tissue.

* Spasm of the artery can be relieved by the use of ..... applied locally.

Papaverine.

* Are there any other ways the artery may be distended if it is still in the state of spasm?

Yes, by injection of saline between two clamps.

* As a last resort, the artery may have to be opened and damaged ..... removed.

Intima.

* The repair to the defect in the artery as a result of surgery might have to involve a ..... patch being applied.

Vein.

Treatment of Established Volkmann's Ischaemic Contracture

Simple exercises might give improved function in ..... cases.

Mild.

In more severe cases, the muscle shortening might be counteracted in two ways. What are they?

1. By shortening the forearm bones.
2. By detachment and distal displacement of the flexor muscle origin.

That is, the muscles which arise from the medial humeral condyle are detached and slid distally enabling the fingers to be ..... .

Extended.

In other severe cases, the dead muscle in front of the forearm might be ..... and a healthy muscle transferred from elsewhere to enable the fingers to be flexed.

Excised.

Give an example of such a tendon transfer to enable finger flexion to take place.

A wrist flexor or wrist extensor of a healthy nature could be transferred to be attached to the tendon of flexor digitorum profundus to enable finger flexion to take place, and a healthy flexor pollicis longus can be used to activate flexion of the digits also.

Name an operation that might stabilise the wrist in a good position.

Arthrodesis of the wrist.

Continuing with the Complications of Supracondylar Fracture of the Humerus

Injury to the Median Nerve

In most cases, the median nerve injury is due to a simple ..... due to pressure on the nerve by the protruding lower end of the ..... fragment.

Neuropraxia.
Proximal.

The treatment, therefore, is usually ..... as the pressure on the nerve is relieved by fracture reduction.

Expectant.

Deformity from Malunion

The commonest deformity to be seen clinically is lateral tilt at the site of the ..... causing a deformity known as ....

Fracture.
Cubitus valgus.

If cubitus valgus has a severe angle, it may be corrected by ..... in the supracondylar region of the humerus.

Osteotomy.

By osteotomy we mean refracturing with a reciprocating saw or osteotome and correcting the ..... .

Alignment.

In this condition of cubitus valgus, the forearm is angled outwards giving rise to some irritation to the nerve on the inner side, namely the ..... nerve.

Ulnar.

Medial tilt of the distal fragment is called ....

Cubitus varus.

Give two further complications of supracondylar fractures.	1. Myositis ossificans.
	2. Elbow stiffness.
* What is this condition of the ulnar nerve called?	Ulnar neuritis.
* Give two manifestations of ulnar neuritis.	1. Weakness of muscles supplied by the ulnar nerve.
	2. Impaired sensation of the skin of the 1½ fingers on the ulnar side of the hand.
* What muscles are supplied by the ulnar nerve in the hand?	1. All the muscles of the hypo-thenar eminence.
	2. All the interossei plus the ulnar two lumbricals.
	3. The adductor of the thumb.

* Volkmann's Ischaemic Contracture

* What is the main feature of this condition?	This is a flexion deformity of the wrist and fingers due to contracture of the flexor muscles in the forearm.
* What is the cause of Volkmann's ischaemic contracture?	Ischaemia of the flexor muscles in the forearm is brought about by obstruction to the brachial artery near the elbow.

Pathology of Volkmann's Ischaemic Contracture

* Does gangrene of the fingers ever follow brachial artery occlusion?	Yes, but very rarely.
* Why does it not happen more often?	Because the collateral circulation is sufficient to keep the hand alive.
* Brachial artery occlusion then involves which muscle groups mainly?	The forearm flexor muscles become ischaemic.
* What happens to the nerves in the forearm?	The peripheral nerve trunks also suffer from ischaemia below the elbow level.
* Name two muscle groups in the forearm that are mainly involved.	1. Flexor digitorum profundus.
	2. Flexor pollicis longus.
* As a result of diminished blood supply, what pathological process takes place in these muscles?	Fibrosis and shortening of the muscles.
* As a result of the ischaemia which nerve trunk is mainly involved?	The median nerve.
* What fractures might cause brachial artery obstruction?	Any fracture in the region of the elbow, e.g. supracondylar fracture in children.
* What produces brachial artery contusion?	The sharp lower end of the main shaft fragment.
* Contusion of the artery causes ..... and ..... in the vessel.	Spasm, thrombosis.
* Name another factor outside the arterial wall that can cause obstruction to the flow of the blood in the artery.	A tight plaster cast or haematoma.

Clinical Features of Volkmann's Ischaemic Contracture

* What is the commonest age group? — Children.

* What is the commonest fracture? — Supracondylar fracture.

* What is the commonest symptom in a child with this condition? — Pain in the forearm.

Physical Examination

* What do the fingers look like in the early stage? — White or blue and cold.

* What happens to the radial pulse? — Absent usually but not always.

* What happens with finger movements? — Weak and painful.

* Passive extension of the fingers is ..... and ..... . — Painful Restricted.

* Would you expect anaesthesia of the fingers and paralysis of the small muscles of the hand in the early stages? — No.

* In the established condition, fixed flexion is seen at which joints? — At the wrist and the finger joints.

* How long after the beginning of the ischaemia does the contracture take place? — A few weeks after the injury.

* What actually produces the flexion deformity? — Shortening of the fibrotic forearm flexor muscles.

* Is the sensory and motor paralysis necessarily a feature of Volkmann's contracture? — No, the contracture is simply the flexion of the wrist and fingers due to shortening of the fibrotic forearm flexor muscles.

* Give two outstanding signs of early Volkmann's contracture. —
  1. Absence of radial pulse.
  2. Unwillingness to extend fingers because of pain.

* Give two further symptoms of early Volkmann's. —
  1. Absence of sensation.
  2. Paralysis of the hand flexor muscles or tender forearm muscles.

* Give three features of Volkmann's ischaemic contracture that are not seen in Dupuytren's contracture. —
  1. In Volkmann's, the wrist is flexed.
  2. All the joints of the fingers are flexed.
  3. In Volkmann's there is no palpable thickening in the palm.

Treatment: Incipient Stage

* How long does it take the changes of brachial artery occlusion to become permanent? — Probably six hours.

* What is the first step in treatment of the incipient stage? — All splints, plaster and bandages are removed and the elbow extended.

* If the fracture is displaced what would you do? — Reduce it.

* If the elbow is dislocated what would you do? — Reduce it.

* How might you produce a dilatation of the vessel that is in spasm, namely the brachial artery? Give two methods.

1. Heat cradle or hot bottles are applied to the other three limbs and trunk to promote general vascular dilatation.
2. Probably preferable to cool affected limb to reduce metabolic needs.

* If these methods fail what would you do?

At operation the brachial artery is explored and if the occlusion is due to kinking or spasm of the artery an attempt is made to relieve it by freeing the vessel and applying Papaverine.

* How else may spasm of the artery be relieved?

By the injection of saline between clamps.

If this fails what might be done as a last resort?

The artery has to be opened and repair effected with a vein patch.

Treatment in Established Cases

* Give two ways in which the muscle shortening might be overcome surgically.

1. By shortening forearm bones.
2. By detachment and distal displacement of flexor muscle origin (muscle slide operation).

Give two muscle transfer operations that might help.

By transferring a wrist flexor or wrist extensor to the tendon of flexor digitorum profundus (after excising the dead muscle) a good result might be obtained.

What about flexor pollicis longus?

This might be motivated also by transferring a wrist flexor or wrist extensor into that tendon.

Is there any place for arthrodesis of the wrist?

Yes, this may be very helpful.

Is there any place for median nerve grafting?

Yes, this might be helpful.

CHAPTER 6

FRACTURE OF THE LOWER END OF THE RADIUS

* What is the other name for this fracture?

Colles' fracture.

* Why is this fracture important?

Because it is the most common fracture seen in practice.

* Is it more common in young adults or in the older age group?

In the older age group.

* Is it more common in men or women?

In women.

* Is it more common in the under 40 age group or over 40 age group?

Over 40 age group.

* How is it produced?

By a fall on the outstretched hand.

* Who was Abraham Colles?

A Dublin surgeon who described the fracture in 1814.

* Is the fracture usually displaced or undisplaced?

It is usually displaced.

* Where is the fracture located?

In the radius within one inch (2.5 cm) of the lower articular surface.

* The lower fragment is displaced in four directions. What are they?

1. The lower fragment is displaced backwards or dorsally.
2. It is displaced laterally or radially.
3. It is tilted backwards.
4. It is driven upwards and impacted into the upper fragment.

* Do we see a vertical extension from time to time into the main fragment?

Yes.

* In what percentage of these fractures is the styloid process fractured?

Fifty percent of cases.

* What is the deformity of Colles' fracture called?

A dinner-fork deformity.

* With this deformity, there is a ..... in the lowest third of the forearm.

Depression.

* Immediately below this depression, there is a marked dorsal prominence due to the distal ....

Fragment being dorsally displaced.

* In what way does the Smith's fracture differ from the Colles' fracture? Give three factors.

1. In the Smith's fracture, the lower fragment is displaced forwards.
2. It is rotated forwards.
3. The articular surface of the lower radius is directed too far anteriorly.

Treatment of Colles' Fractures

* In the process of reducing the fracture, what does one do first of all under general anaesthesia?

Disimpact the fracture.

* In the process of reduction, how are the muscles relaxed?

By general anaesthesia or by regional anaesthesia.

* How is disimpaction achieved?

A longitudinal traction is applied upon the hand and thumb with the elbow held rigidly by an assistant who gives counter traction in this way.

* How do you know when disimpaction has been achieved?

The distal small fragment can be moved freely.

* How is the distal fragment correctly placed?

By applying volarwards or forward pressure over the distal fragment and by pronating the forearm strongly.

* Where is the counter pressure applied?

This is applied in a backward dorsal direction proximal to the fracture.

* Is the wrist held in palmar flexion or in the neutral position?

Neutral position.
Some prefer slight palmar flexion and ulnar deviation with the forearm pronated.

* To digress momentarily, how do you define a Colles' fracture?

A fracture involving the lower radius within one inch of the joint and in fifty percent of cases, the ulnar styloid is fractured.

* Immobilization of the reduced Colles' fracture — give two methods.

1. The complete encircling plaster.
2. The dorsal plaster slab.

* How far does the dorsal plaster slab extend?

On to the dorsum of the forearm and the medial side and the lateral side and from just below elbow to metacarpal necks.

* How is the slab held in position?

By a cotton bandage.

* What is the advantage of the slab?

It allows swelling of the limb after immobilization and can be tightened down repeatedly by reapplying the bandage.

How would you treat swollen blue fingers seen the next day.

Split the bandage immediately.

* Why is it essential to have radiographs taken after one week?

To make certain the fracture has not slipped — a not uncommon event, that requires re-reduction.

* How long is the plaster retained?

Six weeks.

* Is it easy or difficult to re-manipulate two weeks after the fracture was originally straightened?

It is often quite difficult after two weeks.

* Whilst the plaster is on, what exercises would you recommend?

Exercise the fingers, thumb, elbow and shoulder.

Complications of Colles' Fracture

* Name six.

1. Malunion.
2. Subluxation of inferior radio-ulnar joint.
3. Stiffness of fingers.
4. Rupture of extensor pollicis longus tendon.
5. Stiffness of shoulder.
6. Sudeck's atrophy of the bones of the wrist and hand.

Malunion

* Is it correct to say that despite immobilization in plaster, redisplacement may occur during the first week after reduction?

Yes.

* If there is displacement, in which direction do we find the lower radial fragment?

Displaced dorsally, backward and tilted backward.

* What is the main clinical problem with this malunion?

The function of the wrist is impaired.

* Give two ways of treating malunion.

1. Do nothing if the deformity is slight.
2. Re-reduce the fracture by open operation with the aid of an osteotome.

* Once the fracture has been reduced in an open fashion, how would you hold it?

With a screw or Kirschner wire.

* How would you manage the fracture after it has been correctly aligned?

With a plaster cast for six weeks.

Subluxation of the Inferior Radio-ulnar Joint

* How may this be treated surgically?

By excision of the lower end of ulna including its head and about 3 cm of the shaft.

* In the condition of subluxation of inferior radio-ulnar joint, the ulna remains its normal length but what has happened to the radius?

The distal fragment is displaced upwards thus subluxating the radio-ulnar joint.

* What is the commonest symptom?

Pain at the radio-ulnar joint.

* What is noted about the head of the ulna?

It is unduly prominent at the back of the wrist.

* At what level is the head of the ulna seen?

At or even below the level of tip or radial styloid.

* What is the relationship between head of ulna and radial styloid normally?

Always the ulnar head lies proximal to the level of the radial styloid.

Sudeck's Atrophy

* Give three clinical observations that might be made with this condition.

1. Hand and fingers are swollen.
2. Skin is stretched and glossy overlying the joints.
3. The joints become stiff.

* What is a common cause of Sudeck's atrophy?

A Colles' fracture.

* How best is the condition treated?	By elevation of the limb and intense active exercises.
* What is the eventual outcome?	Usually after many months the condition settles.

Rupture of Extensor Pollicis Longus Tendon

* Does this ever occur spontaneously?	Yes.
* Why is extensor pollicis longus more prone to rupture than the other extensor tendons?	Because it takes a sharp bend around Lister's tubercle which, when fractured, can fray the tendon.
* When the tendon is ruptured following Colles' fracture, is it a clean cut or a frayed tendon we see?	A frayed tendon.
* Does the tendon rupture more often after a minor crack fracture or after a Colles' fracture with major displacement?	Surprisingly, after a minor crack fracture it is more common.
* From a clinical point of view, how long after the Colles' fracture might you see rupture of extensor pollicis longus?	Four to eight weeks after the Colles' fracture was sustained.
* On examination, what is the outstanding feature?	Active extension at the inter-phalangeal joint is impossible and extension at the metacarpophalangeal joint is greatly impaired.
* When it comes to treatment, why is end to end anastomosis difficult?	Because of the frayed nature of the tendons.
What operation then would you recommend?	Attach the tendon of extensor indicis to the distal stump of extensor pollicis longus.
* Why does this operation not impair the extensibility of the index finger?	Because the extensor communis tendon supplies the extensor power to the index finger as well as extensor indicis.
What is a Smith's fracture?	A Smith's fracture is a reversed Colles' fracture, i.e. a transverse fracture, just above the wrist with forward displacement of the distal fragment instead of dorsal displacement as in the Colles' fracture.
What is a Barton's fracture?	Barton's fracture is a fracture dislocation in which the distal radius is split longitudinally into ventral and dorsal fragments — the separated ventral fragment shifts proximally carrying the hand with it.
How is it best treated?	Since the fracture is unstable, open reduction and internal fixation using a small anterior plate is recommended.

CHAPTER 7

FRACTURE OF RADIUS AND ULNA

Fracture of the Upper End of the Ulna with Dislocation of the Head of the Radius

What is the other name for this set of circumstances?

Monteggia fracture dislocation.

How is Monteggia fracture sustained? Give two.

1. By forced pronation.
2. By direct blow on the upper ulna.

What happens to the ulna in this injury?

It is fractured and angulated forward in its upper third.

What is the fate of the head of the radius in this set of circumstances?

It is dislocated forwards.

Treatment of Monteggia Fracture

Since the fracture may be produced by forced pronation, how might it be reduced?

By full supination.

If the fracture dislocation is reduced this way, how would you hold the limb in plaster?

With the elbow at a right angle and the forearm fully supinated.

How long would you retain in plaster cast?

Eight weeks.

Is it common or rare for closed reduction to succeed?

Rare, in adults — common in children.

How then would you treat this condition surgically in order to get correct alignment?

The head of the radius is replaced under direct vision and resutured behind the annular ligament. In neglected cases, the head of the radius might be excised.

How would you manage the ulnar fracture?

Through a separate incision along the ulna, reduce the fracture and hold with a plate and screws or a long intramedullary nail.

Is plaster immobilization necessary after this operation?

Yes.

Fractures of the Shaft of the Forearm Bones

Give two ways in which both bones might be fractured.

1. Fall on the hand.
2. Direct blow upon the forearm.

Which muscles attached to the radius may cause additional rotational deformity? Give three.

1. Biceps and supinator in upper third.
2. Pronator teres in middle third.
3. Pronator quadratus in lower third.

Are these fractures easy or difficult to hold correctly reduced?

Difficult.

Are these fractures easy or difficult to hold in children?

Easier than with adults.

45

Why is reduction of a high degree of accuracy essential with these forearm fractures?

Because a slight displacement can cause a malfunction of rotation, that is both pronation and supination may be restricted.

How is the fracture reduced?

With the upper arm held, traction is applied to the fingers with elbow at a right angle and forearm rotated into position.

If one is successful in performing a closed reduction, how would the fracture be held and for how long?

Plaster cast from axilla to metacarpal necks with the elbow at a right angle and the forearm in mid position half way between pronation and supination or in supination with high fracture or in pronation with low fracture. Eight weeks is the period of immobilization.

Why are repeated radiographs at weekly intervals necessary with this fracture?

To make certain it has not slipped within the cast.

How long do these fractures take to unite?

Eight weeks.

Is it common or rare to have to resort to surgery in these fractures?

Common.

How would you proceed to internally fixate these fractures? Would you use one or two incisions?

Obviously two incisions, one for the radius and one for the ulna.

How many screws would each plate have?

Six.

How else might you hold the fracture reduced?

With an intramedullary nail in radius and ulna.

After internal fixation, is plaster required?

Yes.

For how long is it immobilized?

For about twelve weeks.

At what angle is the elbow held?

Ninety degrees.

How do you treat the fracture when the plaster comes off?

With active exercises.

Do all surgeons agree that plaster immobilization is necessary after internal fixation?

No, when the plates are strong, immobilization might not be necessary.

Give three common complications of forearm fractures.

1. Malunion.
2. Delayed union.
3. Non-union.

Give two less common complications of forearm fractures.

1. If compound, osteomyelitis.
2. Arterial occlusion from too tight a plaster.

Un-united fractures may be treated with a Phemister graft that consists of slivers of .... from the ..... .

Cancellous
bone; Ilium.

Where are the slivers placed?

Under the periosteum without disturbing the fracture.

If the position of the un-united fragments is imperfect, what would you recommend?

Perfect the reduction, clear fibrous tissue from both ends of the bone, then graft and plate the fracture.

Apart from plating the ulna, how else may it be internally fixated?

With a long intramedullary nail.

What would you recommend if both bones have established non-union?

Graft each through two separate incisions.

Is it essential to plate the bones after Phemister graft to ulna or radius?

No, internal fixation is not essential but a plaster cast from axilla to metacarpal neck is.

How would you treat non-union in a fracture of the ulna within a centimetre or so of the wrist?

Excise the short distal fragment of ulna.

To what use might the head of ulna be put?

It might be used as a graft if the radius is un-united and requires bone grafting.

Malunion of Forearm Fractures

Give three ways in which function might be impaired with malunion of forearm.

1. Angulation of the fragments.
2. Shortening of one of the bones.
3. Cross union between ulna and radius.

What effect does angulation have on pronation and supination?

It restricts the range of pronation and supination.

What effect does cross union have on pronation and supination?

It renders pronation and supination impossible.

What effect does shortening of one or other bone have on the wrist joint?

It produces subluxation of the inferior radio-ulnar joint.

What effect does subluxation of the wrist joint have? Give two.

1. It gives rise to pain.
2. Restriction of movement.

Is it a common or rare operation to refracture and realign and plate the bones?

This is a rare event.

How may subluxation of inferior radio-ulnar joint be best treated?

By excising the lower end of the ulna.

Fractures of the Shaft of the Radius

When combined with dislocation of the radio-ulnar joint, what name does it take?

Galeazzi fracture dislocation.

Where is the radius fractured?

At the junction of middle and lower third.

How is the Galeazzi fracture sustained?

By a fall on the hand.

What happens to the lower radio-ulnar joint?

The ligaments are ruptured and the head of the ulna is displaced out of the ulnar notch of the radius.

In which direction are the radial fragments angulated?

Toward the ulna.

In which direction may the head of the ulna be shifted? Give three.

1. Medially.
2. Anteriorly or
3. Posteriorly.

To what fracture is the Galeazzi fracture analogous?

Analogous to the Monteggia fracture dislocation in the upper part of the forearm.

Which is more common, the Monteggia or the Galeazzi?

The Galeazzi.

How is the Galeazzi fracture produced and which nerve is commonly involved?

By a fall on the hand — the ulnar nerve.

How is this fracture dislocation best treated?

By open operation and plating of the radius.

What needs to be done about the dislocation of radio-ulnar joint?

Nothing, because when the radius is reduced, so is the radio-ulnar joint.

Is plaster immobilization necessary following this type of internal fixation?

Yes, plaster from axilla to metacarpal necks with the elbow at right angles.

CHAPTER 8

FRACTURES OF THE OLECRANON PROCESS

* How are these fractures sustained?

By a fall on the point of the elbow or by forced flexion of the actively contracted elbow.

* What three forms does the fracture take?

1. A crack without displacement.
2. A clean break with separation into two fragments.
3. A comminuted fracture.

* How would you treat a crack fracture?

Plaster of paris cast for two weeks, for symptomatic treatment only.

Would you have the elbow fully extended or fully flexed?

Flexed to a right angle.

How would you treat a clean fracture with separation?

Open operation is usually indicated, the fracture being reduced perfectly and held by a coarse threaded intramedullary screw or by tension band wiring.

Would you use plaster after this type of internal fixation?

Yes, for three weeks.

Comminuted Fracture of Olecranon Process

Is it possible to re-align these many fragments?

No.

How is this fracture best treated?

Remove all fragments of olecranon and suture triceps to what is left of the ulna.

How are the sutures attached to the ulna?

Through small drill holes.

How long would you immobilize in plaster after this?

Three weeks.

Complications of Fractures of Olecranon Process

* What are the complications of olecranon fractures? Give two.

1. Non-union.
2. Osteoarthritis.

* How would you treat non-union in elderly people?

Do nothing to the fracture and encourage exercises.

* In younger persons, how would you treat an un-united olecranon?

Clean up the fracture surfaces and oppose the two ends and hold with a long screw.

Osteoarthritis of the Olecranon

What treatment would you recommend for this?

Usually nothing has to be done because the symptoms are not severe.

Fracture of the Head of the Radius

* How is this fracture produced?

By a fall on the outstretched hand.

* In what direction is the force transmitted?

Along the shaft of the radius.

* In what percentage of cases is a simple crack seen in the head of the radius?

Fifty percent.

* Of the rest, in what proportion is there a disc shaped wedge displaced from the head of the radius?

More than fifty percent.

* What is the other type of fractured head of radius?

The comminuted fracture.

What is the most outstanding physical sign of fractured head of radius?

Tenderness on palpating the head of the radius.

Which movements would you expect to be painful and restricted?

Pronation and supination.

Radiographs may show one of three features. What are they?

1. Vertical split in radial head.
2. A single fragment broken off.
3. Head broken into several fragments.

* If the initial radiographs fail to show a fracture, is it worthwhile to repeat them taking different angle shots of the head of radius?

Yes, this is most important.

Treatment of Fracture of Head of Radius

* In cases where there is only slight damage, how would you treat it?

Apply a plaster cast with the elbow at a right angle and forearm midway between pronation and supination. Perhaps a sling would suffice.

* How long would you retain the cast?

Three weeks.

* How would you treat the patient after this fracture is united?

With mobilizing exercises.

Treatment in Cases of Severe Damage to Radial Head

* How would you manage this type of fracture?

Total excision of the radial head is advised in order to prevent late osteoarthritis developing.

* Whereabouts is the fracture line in the case of a fracture in this region in childhood?

The neck of the radius.

* How would you treat fracture of the neck of the radius in a child?

By manipulation to correct the position.

* If the neck of the radius is still distorted, how would you manage this case?

By open operation and replacing the head precisely on the neck of the radius.

* Would you ever think of excising the head of the radius in a child?

Never.

* Why would you never excise the head of a radius in a child?

Because as growth occurs, the radius rides up towards the humerus disturbing the relationship with the ulna.

How may a single large fragment be held?

By a Kirschner wire.

Complications of Fracture of the Head of the Radius

* Give two complications.

1. Joint stiffness.
2. Osteoarthritis.

* What is the best treatment for joint stiffness?

Prolonged physiotherapy in the form of heat and exercises.

* What is the usual eventual outcome in cases of joint stiffness?

Most times full recovery is obtained.

* Osteoarthritis: how would you treat established osteoarthritis?

If the head of the radius has not been removed at the time of the accident, then excision of head of radius ought to be undertaken at this time.

* How else would you treat osteoarthritis of the elbow? Give two.

1. Continue with physiotherapy, heat and exercises.
2. Elbow replacement operations are now possible.

CHAPTER 9

SCAPHOID FRACTURE

* In what age group is this commonly seen?

Young adults.

* How is it produced?

Fall on outstretched hand.

* Give one other way that it may be sustained.

By kickback from the starting handle of a motor.

* Where is the commonest site for the fracture of the scaphoid?

Through the middle or the waist.

Give two other less common sites.

1. Proximal pole fracture.
2. Tubercle of scaphoid.

* Are the fragments ever widely displaced?

No.

* What are the main clinical features? Give two.

1. Tenderness in the anatomical snuff box.
2. Fullness in anatomical snuff box.

* What are the four projections you would ask the radiographer to take pictures through in a suspected scaphoid fracture.

1. Antero-posterior projection.
2. Lateral projection.
3. Lateral oblique.
4. Medial oblique.

* If early radiographs are normal, in presence of a likely fracture clinically what would you advise?

Re-radiograph in 10-14 days because the earlier films may not demonstrate the fracture.

Treatment of Fractured Scaphoid

* In standard cases, i.e. waist and proximal pole fractures, how is the fracture immobilized?

In a plaster of paris cast.

* Fow how long is this retained?

Usually up to three months, with two cast changes in that period.

* Since there is no displacement, ... is not required.

Reduction.

* What is the extent of the plaster in fractures of the scaphoid? —

* How far down should the plaster extend?

To the interphalangeal joint of thumb but not including it.

* How far proximally does the cast extend?

To just below the elbow joint.

* Should the metacarpo-phalangeal joint of the thumb be immobilized?

Yes, in the glass holding position.

* Should the thumb be free to move at the inter-phalangeal joint?

Yes.

How would you treat a fracture of scaphoid tubercle?

With crepe bandages and early exercises.

* Complications of Scaphoid Fractures

How may you treat the rare displaced fracture that resists closed reduction.

By open reduction and screw fixation.

Delayed Union

* If bone grafting is decided upon, what method would you use?

Impacting autogenous bone into a deep slot cut in both fragments across the fracture site.

* Are results of bone grafting necessarily successful?

No.

* Is established non-union always painful?

No, sometimes the disability is slight.

Non-union

* Is non-union more or less common with scaphoid fractures than with other fractures?

It is more common.

* What does the scaphoid fracture have in common with sub-capital fractures of the neck of the femur?

Both of these fractures are bathed with synovial fluid since they are intra-articular.

* Give three reasons why the scaphoid fracture may go on to non-union.

1. The fracture line is bathed with synovial fluid preventing a fibrinous bridge forming.
2. Inadequate immobilization.
3. Impairment of the blood supply to proximal fragments giving rise to avascular necrosis of the proximal fragment.

* What are the radiographic appearances of non-union of the scaphoid? Give three.

1. Fracture surfaces become rounded.
2. They become sharply defined as if a joint was forming between them.
3. Cystic changes appear in the proximal sclerosed fragment.

Treatment of Non-union

* Give two explanations for the pain of non-union.

1. Pain from the fracture site.
2. Pain from very early osteoarthritis at the radio-carpal joint.

* Give two methods of treating non-union.

1. Since pain might be slight, some surgeons prefer to take an expectant line.
2. Other surgeons would prefer to do a bone grafting procedure in the hope that the fracture will unite and that osteoarthritis might not develop at the radio-carpal joint.

How may the bone graft be supported?

With a screw and plaster cast.

Avascular Necrosis of Proximal Fragment

* Why is the blood supply of proximal fragment precarious after fractures through the waist or proximal half of the bone?

Because the main nutrient vessel enters the distal end of the distal half of the bone so when the bone is fractured, the blood supply to the proximal fragment is disrupted.

* Does the proximal half of the scaphoid have any other means of obtaining a blood supply?

No, because it does not lie in a vascular bed.

* What is the radiographic appearance of avascular necrosis of the proximal pole of the scaphoid?

The dead or avascular part of the scaphoid looks denser than the rest of the carpal bones.

Treatment of Avascular Necrosis

* What is the usual sequel to leaving the dead bone in situ?

Osteoarthritis of wrist usually develops.

* How might osteoarthritis therefore be avoided?

By excising the dead fragment of scaphoid plus or minus excision of radial styloid.

* If the wrist is still painful and weak following excision of proximal pole, what would you recommend?

Arthrodesis of the wrist.

* Name another procedure that may follow excision of proximal pole.

Replacement of proximal pole with a silicone prosthesis (Silastic).

* What are the long term results of this Silastic implant operation?

Unknown at this point of time.

Osteoarthritis Complicating Fracture of the Scaphoid Bone

* Treatment of osteoarthritis of the wrist is divided into two areas. What are they?

1. If the pain is only slight and the wrist is not used a lot, then a wrist support might do the job.
2. Arthrodesis of the wrist.

* What bones are included in wrist arthrodesis for this condition?

Radio-carpal joint fusion together with inter-carpal fusion (and sparing of the radio-ulnar joint from fusion) is the operation of choice.

Can the wrist be pronated and supinated after this operation?

Yes.

Can the wrist be palmar-flexed and dorsiflexed after this operation?

No.

CHAPTER 10

DISLOCATION OF THE LUNATE BONE

How does this injury take place?

A fall on the outstretched hand.

The hand is extended in the fall, thus enabling the wedge shaped lunate to be squeezed out from between which bones?

The capitate bone and the radius.

The spontaneous reduction of a perilunar dislocation may also dislocate the ..... .

Lunate.

What amount of rotation takes place in the lunate after it has been squeezed out?

It is rotated through ninety degrees and lies in front of the wrist.

The concave surface thus faces ..... .

Forwards.

What major nerve might be injured by this forward rotation of the lunate bone?

Median nerve.

What two clinical features may suggest insufficient room in carpal tunnel.

1. Blunting of sensation in median nerve distribution.
2. Difficulty in flexing the fingers actively.

Treatment

How would you treat a dislocation of the lunate bone?

Apply strong traction in the long axis of the forearm and then apply direct pressure to the front of the wrist. If the lunate goes back apply a cast which is retained for four weeks.

If the manipulation is unsuccessful, what would you recommend?

Open operation and reduction of lunate.

If the dislocation of the lunate has been present for many weeks what would you recommend?

Excision of lunate.

Is the impairment of wrist function slight or gross following excision of lunate?

Gross.

Give three complications of dislocation of the lunate.

1. Avascular necrosis of the lunate.
2. Osteoarthritis of the wrist joint.
3. Injury to median nerve.

How would you diagnose avascular necrosis of the lunate?

The radiograph shows increased density and/or squashing of the bone.

Give two ways of treating avascular necrosis of the lunate.

1. Simple excision of the lunate as early as possible to avoid osteoarthritis.
2. Excision of lunate followed by Silastic prosthesis replacement.

Give two ways of treating osteoarthritis that has followed death of the lunate?

1. Wrist support in mild cases.
2. Arthrodesis of wrist in more severe cases.

How would you treat median nerve compression due to lunate dislocation?

Immediate open reduction of the lunate in early cases and in delayed cases where the lunate has been displaced for several weeks, perhaps excision of lunate is to be considered.

Perilunar Dislocation of the Carpus

In this condition, in what direction does the whole carpus dislocate?

Backwards.

What is the fate of the lunate bone?

It remains in normal relationship with the radius.

In attempting to reduce a perilunar dislocation, what might happen to the lunate bone?

It might become dislocated during the reduction attempt.

If one is unable to reduce a perilunar dislocation with manipulation, what would you recommend?

Operative reduction should be undertaken.

If at operation, the bone is seen to be totally detached, what would you do?

Either excise the lunate or replace it with Silastic.

CHAPTER 11

METACARPAL FRACTURES

* Fracture of the base of the first metacarpal bone. How is it sustained?

A longitudinal blow as in boxing.

* Name two types of fracture of first metacarpal base.

1. A transverse or short oblique fracture across the base of the metacarpal but not entering the joint.
2. An oblique fracture that enters the carpo-metacarpal joint (Bennett's Fracture).

* Why is the Bennett's fracture potentially more dangerous?

Because of the disruption of the adjacent joint, osteoarthritis may develop subsequently.

Treatment of These Two Fractures

How is the Bennett's fracture reduced?

By pulling on long axis of thumb, abducting it and extending it.

There are three ways of holding it — what are they?

1. P.O.P. with felt pad over fracture site.
2. Continuous skin traction with wire splint.
3. Internal fixation with screw or Kirschner wire.

* If closed reduction can't be held with a plaster cast, how would you recommend fixation?

With a small screw or by preventing riding up of the main metacarpal fragment by passing a wire into the adjacent trapezium.

* When these two methods of internal fixation are used, how would you immobilize the fracture of the metacarpal?

With a well fitting plaster cast retained for six weeks and extending up to but not including the elbow.

* Complications of fractures of metacarpal base — Name one.

Osteoarthritis of carpo-metacarpal joint — quite rare.

* How is this prevented?

By accurately reducing and holding reduced with screw or wire in the case of a Bennett's fracture.

* Give two ways of treating established osteoarthritis of the carpo-metacarpal joint.

Excision of trapezium or arthrodesis of the trapezio-metacarpal joint.

Other Fractures of Metacarpal Bones

Give two ways in which metacarpal bones can be fractured.

1. Blow on the knuckle as in boxing.
2. Fall on the hands.

From an anatomical point of view, how would you classify these fractures into three groups?

1. Through the base of the metacarpal bone.
2. Oblique fracture of the shaft.
3. Transverse fracture through the neck of the bone.

Are most of these fractures displaced or undisplaced?

Undisplaced.

How would you treat undisplaced fractures?

Use a dorsal plaster slab for three weeks and encourage exercises of the fingers from the outset.

How would you manage a displaced fracture of a metacarpal neck?

Reduce the fracture by applying traction to the finger and pushing the distal fragment into position, whilst the proximal fragment is held supported. Then hold fracture immobilized with malleable metal strip for three weeks.

If the fracture does not hold well in this position, what would you do?

Internally fixate it with an intramedullary wire.

Would you introduce the intramedullary wire from the distal end or the proximal end?

From the proximal end, thus sparing the metacarpo-phalangeal joint from encroachment.

If volar angulation is less than 40 degrees is resultant disability gross or slight?

Slight.

CHAPTER 12

PHALANGEAL FRACTURES

* Classify fractures of the phalanges into four groups.

1. Long spiral fracture of shaft.
2. Oblique fracture.
3. Transverse fracture.
4. Comminuted fracture of distal phalanx.

How are they usually sustained?

By direct violence.

Treatment of Phalangeal Fractures

* Why is protracted immobilization of a finger beyond two weeks unwise?

The finger joints may stiffen in the position of immobilization thus losing flexion and extension.

* Do phalangeal fractures ever go on to non-union?

No, very rarely.

* Why then does one splint these fractures? Give two reasons.

1. To prevent redisplacement if they have required reduction.
2. To relieve pain.

* Since the fractures are painless and well on the way to union by the second or third week, ... should be commenced after the second or third week.

Mobilizing exercises.

* How would you treat a comminuted fracture of phalanx?

Reduce fracture with manipulation under anaesthesia and then hold finger semi-flexed with an aluminium splint for two weeks.

How else may the fracture be held?

With rolled bandage in palm, fractured finger is held flexed by another crepe bandage.

* If the phalanx can't be reduced this way, how should you do it?

Open operation and internal fixation with an intramedullary wire.

CHAPTER 13

MALLET FINGER

* What is the other name for a mallet finger?

Baseball finger.

What tendon is involved in this injury?

The extensor tendon to the terminal phalanx.

* How is this injury produced? Give two methods.

1. A sudden injury in which the end of the finger is forcibly extended during acute flexion and snaps the tendon or avulses a small part of the terminal phalanx to which the extensor tendon is attached.
2. A sharp knife may readily divide the extensor tendon producing a mallet finger.

* What is the patient's main complaint?

Inability to extend the distal interphalangeal joint.

* In the treatment of this condition, how is the finger held?

The finger should be immobilized for three weeks with the proximal interphalangeal joint flexed and the distal interphalangeal joint held in neutral position with an intramedullary wire or with a zimmer splint.

* If there is wide separation between the bone fragment and the bed of the bone, what treatment would you recommend?

Open operation and suturing of avulsed bone to the bed at the proximal end of the distal phalanx.

* How would you manage neglected and unsuccessfully treated cases of mallet finger?

Most patients would accept an inability to extend terminal phalanx through twenty or thirty degrees and would, therefore, feel nothing should be done.

* If something had to be done to correct this lack of extension, what would you recommend?

Excision of about two millimetres of the extensor tendon over the middle phalanx and suture the two remaining ends together and then hold the terminal phalanx fully extended with an intramedullary wire up the pulp of the finger.

* How would you manage a mallet finger due to a lacerated extensor tendon?

The sooner the two ends of the tendon are sutured, the better is the result. After joining the two ends, the finger is held in the neutral position for six weeks with the aid of an intramedullary wire.

CHAPTER 14

FRACTURES OF THE PELVIS AND ASSOCIATED BLADDER, URETHRAL AND SCIATIC NERVE INJURIES

Fractures of the Pelvis

Classify fractures of the pelvis into two groups.

1. Isolated fractures not destroying the integrity of the pelvic ring.
2. Fractures with disruption of the pelvic ring.

Give examples of isolated fractures not destroying the integrity of the pelvic ring. Give five.

1. Fracture of the superior ischio pubic ramus.
2. Fractures of the inferior ischio pubic ramus.
3. Fractures entering the acetabulum.
4. Fracture of wing of ilium.
5. Avulsion of anterior, superior iliac spine or anterior, inferior iliac spine.

In the diagnosis of pelvic fractures, name the four essential radiographic views that should be taken.

1. Anteroposterior.
2. Inlet view with tube tilted 20-30 Deg caudad.
3. & 4. Right and left oblique views.

Isolated Fractures

Name four muscles whose violent contraction may avulse a part of the pelvis.

1. Sartorius – Anterior Superior Iliac Spine.
2. Rectus Femoris – Anterior Inferior Iliac Spine.
3. Adductor Longus – Pubic Bone.
4. Hamstrings – part of Ischium.

How would you treat these isolated fractures, the commonest being of the superior or inferior ischio pubic ramus?

No special treatment is needed; rest in bed for two to three weeks is sufficient.

Fractures with Disruption of the Pelvic Ring

What bones constitute the pelvic ring?

The sacrum.
The two innominate bones.

Give three mechanisms of ring fractures.

1. Antero-Posterior Compression fracturing both pubic rami.
2. Hinge Force – Run over patient has one blade of ilium opened.
3. Fall on one leg causes upward displacement of pubis and ilium on same side.

Since these bones constitute a ring, a fracture must take place at two ..... opposite each other.

Points.

Give two possible sites then for the anteriorly placed injury of the pelvic ring.

1. Fracture through ischio pubic rami or
2. Disruption of symphysis pubis.

Where is the posterior injury in the pelvic ring? Give three.	1. Subluxation of the sacroiliac joint.
	2. Fracture through the ilium.
	3. Fracture through the lateral mass of the sacrum near the sacroiliac joint.

Treatment

If the displacement is slight, how would you treat these disrupted pelvic ring fractures? E.g. Antero-Posterior compression fracture.	Four to six weeks of bed rest is usually adequate.
If there is wide disruption of symphysis pubis, how would you treat this?	Reduction should be performed in the following manner: Apply a short hip spica well padded and extending down to just above one knee. When it is dry, remove a strip 4 cm. wide from the front. Wind an esmarch rubber bandage around the plaster jacket till the gap in the front is closed. As the rubber applies tension, the gap in the front is closed and the separation of symphysis pubis gradually reduces.
For how long should this plaster be retained?	Four weeks.
Give an alternative method of reducing and holding reduced a separated symphysis pubis.	Wire or plate and four screws can be applied to the pubic bone after reduction which may also be achieved with a pelvic sling.
How would you reduce a fracture that has resulted in upward displacement of half the pelvis?	Reduce this displacement by applying traction through a tibial pin. Retain traction for six weeks.

Complications of Pelvic Fractures

Give six.	1. Rupture of bladder.
	2. Rupture of urethra.
	3. Rupture of rectum.
	4. Injury to major blood vessel.
	5. Injury to nerves.
	6. Involvement of acetabulum giving rise to osteoarthritis in later life.
If the patient cannot pass urine, why avoid catheterisation?	Because urethrography is less harmful and will show a urethral tear.
Rupture of the bladder. Is this usually extra-peritoneal or intra-peritoneal?	Extra-peritoneal.
Therefore, whither does the urine escape?	Into the perivesical space.
What happens when you pass a catheter?	The bladder is found to be empty.
Give the three principles of treatment.	1. Urgent operation by a urologist should secure suturing of the rent.
	2. Drainage of the bladder.
	3. Drainage of the perivesical space.

Rupture of the Urethra

Which fracture of pelvis usually causes it?   Diastasis of symphysis pubis.

What part of the urethra is involved or ruptured?   Membranous urethra.

Whither does the urine flow?   Into the perineum.

How is the diagnosis confirmed?
1. By inability to pass a catheter into the bladder.
2. By urethrogram.

Treatment of Rupture of Urethra

Whose assistance would you seek for emergency surgery here?   That of a urologist.

The two ends of the urethra have to be sought and this is done through what incision?   Through an incision in the perineum.

How does one suture the ends together accurately?   Over a catheter.

How is the bladder rested whilst the urethra is healing?   By means of a supra pubic drain in the bladder.

Injury to rectum — is this rare or common?   It is rare.

Injury to major blood vessel — is this rare or common?   It is rare.

What vessel might be ruptured?   The common iliac artery might be damaged by a spicule of bone.

Give two ways of treating this.
1. By suturing the rent.
2. By vein graft.

If a small vessel was ruptured, how would you treat that?   By ligation of the small vessel.

For example, if the superior gluteal artery was severed, what measures might we take to stop the haemorrhage?   Ligation of the internal iliac artery proximal to the superior gluteal branch.

Injury to Nerves

With major disruption of the pelvic ring — are nerve injuries common or rare?   Injury to lumbo-sacral plexus is common.

Are these nerve injuries irrecoverable or otherwise?   They are usually irrecoverable.

What is the complication of a fracture involving the acetabulum?   Osteoarthritis of the hip joint in later life.

Fractures of the Acetabulum

Name the four major types of Acetabulum Fracture.

1. Anterior Pillar.
2. Posterior Pillar.
3. Transverse Fracture — usually just above cotyloid notch.
4. Composite Fracture.

Which two may damage the weight bearing surface thus producing post-traumatic osteoarthritis?

1. Transverse.
2. Composite (always).

Name two types of injury that may fracture the Acetabulum.

1. Traffic accident.
2. Fall from a height.

Name three common associated fractures.

Fractures of: 1. Knee.
2. Femur.
3. Calcaneum.

What are the three views that should be taken by the radiographer?

1. Standard antero-posterior.
2. Pelvic inlet, i.e. wth tube tilted 20-30 deg. caudad.
3. The two obliques at 45 degrees.

Give the two features of emergency treatment.

1. Replace lost blood.
2. Reduce a dislocation with 10 kg of traction.

Treatment of Anterior and Posterior Fractures

If traction has afforded good reduction, what would you do?

Continue with traction for eight weeks.

If position unacceptable, what then?

Internally fixate with lag screw or compression plate.

Through which approach would you intervene?

1. Smith-Peterson for anterior fractures.
2. 'Southern' approach for posterior fractures.

Severely comminuted fractures are best treated .....Ultimately, a painful stiff arthritic hip may

Conservatively, with continued traction until union is established.
Arthroplasty.

require ..... .

CHAPTER 15

FRACTURE OF THE NECK OF THE FEMUR

* What three types of fractures do you recognise?

1. Subcapital.
2. Mid cervical.
3. Pertrochanteric.

* Where is the fracture line in a subcapital fracture?

Immediately inferior to the head of the femur.

* Where is the fracture line in a mid cervical fracture?

The fracture line is about the middle of the neck of the femur.

* Where is the fracture line in a pertrochanteric type of fractured neck of femur?

The fracture line runs from the greater trochanter to the lesser trochanter.

* What are the other names for pertrochanteric fractures?

Inter-trochanteric or simply trochanteric.

* Which of these three fractures is considered the most serious?

Subcapital.

* Why is the subcapital the most serious?

Because it has the most complications.

* What are they (3)?

1. Non-union.
2. Avascular necrosis of head of femur.
3. Late osteoarthritis.

* Most patients are over ..... years of age.

Sixty.

* Most patients with this type of fracture are of the ..... sex.

Female.

* How are these fractured necks of femora produced?

Usually by a fall or stumble and frequently there is a rotational force as well.

* In 95% of cases, there is displacement. What displacement?

The shaft fragment is markedly rotated laterally and is displaced proximally.

* If the shaft fragment is rotated laterally, this means the foot of the patient is seen to be turned ..... .

Outward.

* If the shaft fragment is displaced upwards, this means the limb is ..... than its fellow.

Shorter.

If in Casualty then we see an elderly lady with her foot turned outward and the limb shorter than the other one, she quite possibly has suffered a ....

Fractured neck of femur.

* If the shaft fragment is rotated laterally and displaced upwards, this means we are dealing with a ..... fracture of neck of the femur.

Displaced.

* What percentage of fractured necks of femur are of the displaced variety?

Ninety-five percent.

* What name is given to those fractured necks that are not displaced?

These are called impacted fractures of the neck of the femur.

* With impacted fractures, is the limb abducted or adducted?

Abducted.

Clinical Features

* These are composed of symptoms and signs:

* What are the symptoms?

The patient usually describes a trip or stumble which resulted in falling to the ground and being unable to get up again and walk. There is much pain.

* What are the signs?

The foot is turned outward or externally rotated as a result of the shaft fragment being rotated laterally. The limb is shortened by as much as an inch or so due to the proximal displacement of the shaft fragment.

* What is the other name for the impacted fracture?

Impacted abduction fracture.

What are the clinical features (symptoms and signs) with the rare impacted fracture?

Symptoms — patient may have been able to get up after the fall and on occasions, they have been able to walk a short distance in spite of groin pain. *Signs* — there is no evidence of shortening or external rotation as with the displaced fracture, but pain in the groin is a feature.

* How is the diagnosis of fractured neck of femur clinched?

With the aid of the radiograph.

Treatment of Subcapital and Mid Cervical Fractures of Neck of Femur

Displaced fractures.

* In the standard method, what is the name of the three flanged pin used to hold the fragments together?

Smith-Petersen pin.

Name two alternative fixation methods, that nowadays enjoy greater popularity.

1. Sliding Zimmer or Richards screw with plate.
2. Multiple lag screws.

* What do the Smith-Petersen pin and the sliding screw have down their centres?

A hole.

* What is its purpose?

This is to enable the pin or screw to be passed over a guide wire.

* What is the purpose of the guide wire?

This is to guide the pin or screw across the fracture site at the correct level.

Both the Richards and Zimmer screws have a sliding device — what is its purpose?

It permits compression or impaction at the fracture site without the risk of the screw penetrating the acetabulum.

* After the guide wire has been driven across the fracture site, how does one ascertain that its position is satisfactory?

With the aid of radiographs or X-rays taken in two planes, or with aid of an image intensifier.

* When the guide wire has been correctly placed, what is the next step?

To drive the Smith-Petersen pin or screw over the guide wire and thus across the fracture site.

* Upon what type of table is this pinning carried out?

Orthopaedic table.

* What type of anaesthetic is the patient given?

General, usually or spinal if patient has poor respiratory function.

* Before pinning the fracture, it must be ..... .

Reduced.

* How is reduction effected?

Since the leg is externally rotated and shortened, then to reduce the fracture one must internally rotate and pull in the long axis of the leg in order to restore length.

* Are splints required after the patient has been returned to bed following this operation?

No. Free hip movements are encouraged immediately after this operation.

* When does the patient bear weight on the limb following this operation?

At one week post operatively, in most cases.

* Name an alternative method of treatment for the subcapital fracture of the neck of the femur.

Moore's or Thompson's prosthesis: some surgeons when dealing with elderly patients proceed directly to the excision of the head fragment and the replacement of it by means of a metal head. This is called hemiarthroplasty.

* Why is femoral head replacement recommended?

Because the subcapital fracture has a high non-union rate and replacement arthroplasty allows early ambulation some three or four days post-operatively. If the subcapital fracture is pinned, then in fifty percent of patients over the age of sixty years a second operation will have to be undertaken due to non-union. Early hip replacement then avoids that second operation.

* Is it necessary to pin an impacted abduction fracture?

No. The bones are compressed one into the other and usually this gives sufficient rigidity at the fracture site to render internal fixation unnecessary.

* How are these patients with impacted abduction fractures treated?

By means of simple Russell traction which holds the limb suspended in a comfortable position.

* How long is this Russell traction maintained?

Four weeks or so.

* When dealing with the impacted fracture, when is weight bearing permitted?

Six weeks after the injury was sustained.

Complications of Subcapital and Mid Cervical Fractures of the Neck of the Femur

Give four general complications seen in elderly patients with these fractures.

1. Deep vein thrombosis.
2. Pulmonary embolus.
3. Pneumonia.
4. Bedsores.

* Name three specific complications.

1. Non-union.
2. Avascular necrosis.
3. Late osteoarthritis.

* What percentage of subcapital fractures in the elderly proceed to non-union?

Fifty percent.

* What are the causes of non-union?

1. Inadequate blood supply to the femoral head with consequent avascular necrosis.
2. Incomplete immobilization.
3. Flushing of the fracture haematoma by synovial fluid.

Of what significance is an unduly vertical fracture line?

Non-union is more likely.

* What is the commonest cause of non-union?

Avascular necrosis.

* Considering avascular necrosis, what are the three routes of blood supply to the femoral head?

1. The vessels in the ligamentum teres.
2. The capsular vessels that pass up the femoral neck.
3. Branches of the nutrient vessels within the substance of the bones.

In what percentage of adults may 1. above be absent or small?

20%.

* Routes 2 and 3 described are likely to be cut off in a ..... fracture.

Subcapital.

What may be the first indication of necrosis?

Extrusion of nail.

* What are the consequences of non-union?

The symptoms and signs of the original fracture are to be seen again. Furthermore, the Smith-Petersen pin frequently extrudes.

* What are these symptoms and signs?

The groin becomes painful and the limb falls into lateral rotation and shortening is also a feature.

How long may increased X-ray density take to become apparent?

Many months.

* Give three methods of dealing with non-union in the elderly.

1. Replacement arthroplasty of the hip (e.g. Moore's or Thompson's prostheses).
2. Simple removal of the pin without further treatment is indicated in the elderly plus a raised heel and a stick.
3. Excision arthroplasty of the hip may be carried out in the elderly, i.e. Girdlestone's arthroplasty which is simple removal of the head.

In the relatively young what may be done?

1. Subtrochanteric osteotomy to make fracture line more horizontal.
2. If fracture was poorly reduced, remove nail, re-reduce and re-nail correctly and add a fibular graft.
3. If head avascular, replace with metal prosthesis.

* Which of these three operations is the one most commonly used?

Replacement arthroplasty. That is, the head is excised and replaced by a metal prosthesis known as a Moore's or Thompson's prosthesis.

Is there a place for total joint replacement?

Yes, some surgeons prefer to replace both acetabulum and femoral head.

Fractures of the Trochanteric Region of the Neck of the Femur

* What is meant by a trochanteric fracture?

This term is used to describe any fracture in the region that lies approximately between the greater and lesser trochanter.

* Do trochanteric fractures have a better or worse prognosis than subcapital fractures?

Better because they almost invariably unite without complications.

* With trochanteric fractures, what additional metal is used to ensure rigid immobilization at the fracture site?

A plate and screws are attached to the Smith-Petersen pin or Thornton pin, or a one piece pin and plate may be used, e.g. Jewitt.

* Name two stronger fixation devices used in these fractures.

1. A.O. Blade Plate.
2. Sliding Zimmer or Richards Screw and Plate.

* Do these fractures unite more or less readily than other neck fractures?

More readily.

* Are trochanteric fractures prone to complications?

No, they are not as prone to complications as subcapital fractures.

* Are they commoner in men or women?

Women.

* Are they more common in the younger or older age group?

Usually after the age of seventy-five years. The symptoms are almost identical with those of a fractured neck of femur.

* What are the two outstanding physical signs?

External rotation of the limb and shortening.

* Since the fracture is outside the joint capsule, where would you expect the bruising to be seen?

Ecchymosis appears on the back of the upper thigh.

* With mid cervical or subcapital fractures, where is the bruising?

There is none because the blood is retained within the capsule.

The leg is shorter and more externally rotated with these fractures than with subcapital — true or false?

True.

Can the patient lift her leg?

No.

* How is the diagnosis of trochanteric fracture clinched?

By radiography in two planes.

Treatment of Fractures of Trochanteric Region

* Why is surgical intervention preferred to conservative treatment?

Because the patient can enjoy early mobility following internal fixation of the fracture.

* What sort of internal fixation is usually used?

A pin and plate, that is, a Smith-Petersen pin and plate, Thornton pin and plate, or Jewitt pin plate or a Blade plate, or a screw/plate combination, or Ender's nails.

69

* Where is the pin driven?	Up the neck of the femur.
* Where are the screws placed?	Through holes in the plate and then across the shaft of the femur through lateral and medial cortices.
What is the significance of separation of lesser trochanter?	The fracture is unstable and so delay weight bearing.

Some Points of Technique of Internal Fixation of the Trochanteric Fracture

How is the fracture reduced?	By applying traction and medial rotation after the patient is anaesthetised and on the operating table.
How is the appropriate position of the pin ascertained?	By passing a guide wire up the neck of the femur.
How is the position of the guide wire checked?	With radiographs in two planes or image intensifier.
When the guide wire is seen to be perfectly placed, what is the next step?	The driving of a triflanged pin or screwing a large threaded screw (cannulated) over the guide wire.
A plate is then attached to the triflanged pin by means of a ..... and screws are driven through holes in the plate across to the ..... of the medial side of the upper femur.	Screw. Cortex.
Following this operation, is traction needed?	No.
Through what part of the femur are Ender's nails inserted?	Medial femoral condyle.
When is the patient allowed out of bed?	Within two or three days non-weight bearing on crutches is permitted.
Under what circumstances would you use conservative measures for the treatment of fractures of the trochanteric region of the femur? Give three.	1. Some surgeons would treat young patients conservatively since they feel operation is meddlesome because the fracture always unites. 2. If the patient refuses operation, then traction is applied. 3. If patient is too unfit for operation.
* Give the name of the traction that is most suitable for this type of fracture.	Hamilton Russell traction is used.
For how long would the traction be applied?	Ten-twelve weeks.

A Further Method of Treating Trochanteric Fracture

Under what circumstances would you recommend a plaster spica to be used in the treatment of trochanteric fractures?	Occasionally in children.

Complications of Trochanteric Fractures

What is the commonest complication?	Mal-union.

What is the commonest mal-union deformity?	Coxa vara (reduced neck/shaft angle).
Is coxa vara associated with shortening?	Yes.
How would you treat slight shortening that followed trochanteric fracture?	A build up to the heel on the affected side.

Fractures of the Neck of the Femur

Further questions:

* Are fractures of the neck of the femur commoner in persons over sixty years or under sixty years?	Over sixty years.
* Name a condition that predisposes to fracture of femoral neck.	Generalized osteoporosis.
* Since the fracture takes place through a weakened bone, the fracture might well be classified as a ..... fracture.	Pathological.
* The causative force is often	Slight.
* Is the fracture caused by a rotational force or a direct force in most cases?	By a rotational force.
* Is it a small or large percentage of patients who manifest marked displacement with lateral rotation of the limb?	In over ninety percent of cases, there is marked lateral rotation and upward displacement of the involved limb.
* What happens in those fractures that are not markedly displaced? Are they impacted or disimpacted?	Impacted.
* What is meant by impacted?	The two fragments, namely the head and the neck, are jammed in one upon the other.
* With the impacted fracture, there is usually slight ..... of the distal fragment upon the proximal.	Abduction.
* This fracture then is known as impacted ..... fracture.	Abduction.

Clinical Features of Fractures of the Neck of the Femur

* The patient is usually an elderly woman with a story of having tripped and was unable to take ..... on the limb.	Weight.
* Physical examination shows two very common features when simply looking at the injured lower limb. What are they?	1. Marked lateral rotation of the limb. 2. Shortening of the limb.
* The rotation is such that the foot instead of pointing up to the ceiling like the good one, is pointing at ..... degrees to the vertical.	Ninety.
* Likewise, the patella points	Laterally.
* The limb as a whole is ..... by about two or three centimetres.	Shortened.

* Movement of the hip causes	Severe pain.
* In the rare impacted abduction fracture, the pain is much ..... and the patient can often ..... on the injured limb.	Less. Walk.
* Give three ways in which the rare impacted abduction fracture differs from the more common fracture of the neck of the femur.	1. The impacted fracture shows no detectable shortening. 2. The impacted fracture shows no rotational deformity. 3. The hip can be moved through a moderate range without severe pain in the impacted fracture.

Radiographic Examination of the Fractured Neck of Femur

* Do the radiographs show an obvious fracture in all cases of impacted abduction fracture?	No. Often the fracture is barely discernible on the radiograph.
* If there be any doubts, then a ..... radiograph is essential for diagnosis in these cases.	Lateral.
* How else may the diagnosis be made?	By means of a bone scan.

Treatment of the Fractures of the Neck of the Femur

* Displaced fractures and impacted abduction fractures are considered separately.

Displaced Fractures of the Neck of the Femur

* The accepted treatment is to fix the fragments ..... by a suitable metal device.	Internally.
* The triflanged pin, called the .... pin has been used for many years, but the most modern concept is to use a .... in conjunction with a	Smith-Petersen. Compression Screw. Plate.

Technique of Internal Fixation for Femoral Neck Fractures

* How is the fracture reduced?	By carrying out the reversal of the deforming force so the limb is medially or internally rotated and traction is applied in the line of the femur. In this way, the external rotation and shortening are both overcome and the fracture reduced.
During the process of internal fixation, the above procedure is carried out on an orthopaedic table and once reduced, the fracture is maintained in the correct position by binding the foot to a .... which is part of the orthopaedic table.	Foot plate.
How does one confirm that the fracture has been adequately reduced?	By antero-posterior and lateral radiographs, or by means of a television-monitored image intensifier.

How is the triflanged pin or screw placed in the correct position?

By means of a guide wire that is driven across the fracture site.

The position of the guide wire is, of course, confirmed to be correct with the aid of the abovementioned radiographs or ....

Image intensifier.

When antero-posterior and lateral radiographs confirm that the guide wire is in the correct position, the triflanged pin is then driven over the correctly placed ....

Guide wire.

Clearly, the triflanged pin has a central cannula or hole that enables it to be slipped over the correctly-placed guide wire. How is the screw that is placed above the Smith-Petersen pin located?

Again, this is with a guide wire placed 1.25 cm. above the Smith-Petersen pin.

After the pin and screw or pin plate have been correctly inserted and the wound closed, is. it necessary to immobilize the patient in bed?

No, the patient can be left free in bed without any traction device.

For how long would you recommend that the patient refrain from taking weight on the involved limb after internal fixation?

Three months.

With very elderly patients who have difficulty using crutches and non-weight bearing on one limb, some surgeons permit early mobilization with a little weight bearing within the first week or two after surgery.

Give four ways in which a pertrochanteric fracture may be immobilized.

1. Smith-Petersen pin and plate or Thornton pin and plate.
2. Jewitt one piece pin and plate.
3. Sliding screw/plate (Zimmer or Richards).
4. Blade plate (A.O.).

Subcapital Fractures of the Neck of the Femur Alternative Methods for Special Cases

Since pinning does not always succeed, many surgeons perform immediate ..... of the femoral head and it is then replaced by a ....

Excision.
Metal prosthesis.

Is this method common or rare?

Common.

The excision of the fractured head and its replacement with a metal head is called a replacement ....

Hemi arthroplasty.

Sometimes in addition to replacing the head, the acetabulum is replaced also with a plastic socket and this operation is known as ....

Total replacement
Arthroplasty.

When would one decide to do a total replacement arthroplasty?

When the bones are very soft or the joint arthritic.

Replacement arthroplasty then is recommended for people over the age of ..... and for people whose fracture is of the ..... type.

Seventy.
Subcapital.

Treatment of Fractured Neck of Femur in Children

Give two methods of treatment of fractured necks of femur in children?

1. By insertion of two or three threaded pins after manipulative reduction.
2. By manipulative reduction and immobilization in plaster spica.

Impacted Abduction Fractures

These fractures should be treated ..... .

Conservatively.

By this is meant a period of ..... weeks in bed and during this time, the hip and knee are to be exercised.

Three.

After three weeks, partial weight-bearing can be commenced with the aid of crutches. When would full weight-bearing be permitted with an impacted abduction fracture?

At about the eighth week.

Some patients might feel happier about internally fixating .... fractures. The conservative method mentioned above, however, is to be preferred.

Impacted abduction.

Give the three main features of an impacted abduction fracture from a clinical point of view.

1. The hip joint can be moved with only slight pain.
2. There is no shortening.
3. There is no external rotation.

Complications of Fractures of the Neck of the Femur

Give three complications.

1. Avascular necrosis.
2. Non-union.
3. Late osteoarthritis.

Are these three complications more often seen in impacted fractures or in fractures with displacement?

In fractures with displacement.

Avascular Necrosis

The blood supply to the femoral head comes from three sources. What are they?

1. Through the artery to the ligamentum teres.
2. Through the capsular vessels in the femoral neck.
3. Through branches of the nutrient vessels.

When the neck of the femur is fractured, which vessels are severed?

Nutrient and capsular vessels.

What is the significance of a high fracture of the neck of the femur?

The higher the fracture, the more complete is the interruption of these blood vessels.

With higher fractures, then the blood supply to the head might come solely from the artery to the ligamentum teres and this is frequently ..... in elderly people.

Inadequate.

As a result of the inadequate blood supply, the bone cells ..... and this is known as avascular ....

Die.
Necrosis.

If the bone cells are dead, of course, the fracture may fail to ..... .

Unite.

The diminished blood supply to the head may give rise to the degenerative change known as ....

Osteoarthritis.

Give three consequences then of avascular necrosis.

1. Non-union of the fracture.
2. Degenerative arthritis.
3. Complete collapse of the femoral head.

Non-union of Fractures of the Neck of the Femur

In what percentage of cases of subcapital fractures does this happen in people over sixty?

Fifty percent.

Give three causes of non-union of these fractures.

1. Inadequate blood supply giving rise to avascular necrosis.
2. Incomplete immobilization.
3. Flushing of the fracture haematoma by synovial fluid.

Name the commonest causes of incomplete immobilization.

Insertion of a badly-placed pin in a poorly reduced fracture.

Why is flushing of the fracture haematoma by synovial fluid, a factor in this particular type of fracture?

Because the fracture is intra-capsular.

If the synovial fluid washes away the haematoma, then the process of new bone formation cannot take place.

When non-union takes place, what happens to the pin that has been placed across the fracture site?

It tends to back out.

What happens to the head at the same time?

The femoral head sinks down towards the trochanter.

Give four features that the patient would notice with non-union.

1. Recurrence of hip pain.
2. Shortening of the limb as a whole.
3. External rotation of the involved limb.
4. Inability to walk.

How long after the pinning operation would one expect to see these clinical features of non-union?

Anywhere between a few weeks to three years.

Treatment of Non-union of Fractures of the Neck of the Femur

* Give three methods that can be used in the treatment of non-union.

1. Replacement arthroplasty of the hip (Moore's or Thompson's prostheses).
2. Simple removal of the pin without further treatment in elderly patients.
3. Excision arthroplasty of the hip in elderly patients.

* Of these three operations, which is the commonest to be advocated?

Prosthetic replacement of the femoral head alone.

How may a Thompson's prosthesis be anchored in the femoral canal?

With bone cement.

Of what is the cement made?

Acrylic i.e., Methylmethacrylate.

What is the main advantage with a Moore's or Thompson's prosthesis insertion?

Full weight-bearing may be commenced two days post-operatively in most cases.

When would one do a total replacement arthroplasty?

Only when the acetabulum is disorganized or roughened, as in osteoarthritis.

Total replacement arthroplasty implies the insertion of an acetabular .... as well as a femoral stainless steel head.

Plastic cup.

Give one complication of half-joint replacement arthroplasty.

Erosion of the acetabulum sometimes occurs giving rise to medial migration of the prosthetic femoral head.

Excision Arthroplasty. What is the other name for this?

Girdlestone pseudarthrosis.

How is this operation performed?

The head and neck of the femur are excised and the gluteus medius muscle sutured into the acetabulum, the upper half of which is removed.

When is this operation indicated?

As a salvage procedure when a Thompson's or Moore's has failed due to infection or other causes.

Osteoarthritis as a Complication of Fractured Neck of Femur

Give three reasons for this development.

1. Mechanical damage to the articular cartilage at the time of fracture.
2. Impairment of blood supply following the fracture.
3. When union has taken place with faulty alignment.

The commonest operative way of treating osteoarthritis is by ....

Total hip joint replacement.

CHAPTER 16

FRACTURES OF THE SHAFT OF THE FEMUR

* What is the commonest age for fractured shafts of femur?

Any age.

* What is the nature of the violence?

Motor cycle accident or other violent form of injury.

How is a spiral fracture caused?

By a twisting force with the foot anchored.

* Is the fracture as common in the upper third as it is in the lower third?

Yes.

* Give four types of fractures of the shaft of femur.

1. Transverse.
2. Oblique.
3. Spiral.
4. Comminuted (Greenstick in children).

Which is the most common site?

The middle third.

* Metastatic fractures are commoner in the upper third or the lower third?

Upper third.

Why should pelvic radiographs be taken?

To avoid missing a hip or pelvis injury.

* Conservative treatment:

At the site of accident what should be done?

1. Treat the shock.
2. Splint the fracture.

* With conservative treatment, how is the fracture reduced? Give two means.

1. By traction.
2. By manipulation.

With open fractures avoid ....

Internal fixation.

* How is the limb supported?

In a Thomas' splint.

* How is the traction and reduction maintained?

By weights attached to a traction device.

* How is the traction device attached to the leg? Give two ways.

1. By adhesive strapping attached to the skin.
2. By a Steinmann pin through the upper end of the tibia.

What is the main drawback with closed treatment?

The time spent in bed.

* When the limb is in the Thomas' splint, how is the knee flexion arranged?

With a Pearson knee flexion attachment.

* Is an anaesthetic necessary for the reduction?

Not always.

* What stops the limb falling through between the bars of the Thomas' splint?

Canvas slings that are attached to the two metal bars.

What type of embolus commonly complicates the picture?

Fat.

How may the patient be mobilized earlier with closed treatment?

With functional bracing.

Is this treatment more suitable for upper or lower half fractures?

Lower half.

* Give an approximation as to what poundage would be necessary to hold a fractured femur in the corrected position.

Fifteen-twenty pounds.

* How long does union take in most cases of shaft fractures?

Ten-fourteen weeks.

* How is the Thomas' splint suspended above the bed?

By means of a balanced weight technique. The Thomas' splint is attached to an overhead beam.

* What degree of flexion is applied to the knee?

Fifteen-twenty degrees.

Is there any alternative to the Thomas splint?

Yes, some prefer to support the limb on a pillow.

Rehabilitation

* About one week after the fracture, mobilizing exercises are commenced to which joints? Give three.

1. Ankle joint.
2. Knee joint.
3. Hip joint.

* The knee can be placed through how many degrees of flexion with safety during this prolonged traction period?

Sixty degrees.

* How much extension would be recommended at the knee joint whilst in traction?

Full extension is permitted and desirable in order to prevent a flexion deformity at the knee.

* What about ankle movement?

Both plantar flexion and dorsi flexion should be encouraged immediately.

* What is the average duration of traction necessary to see firm union established?

About twelve weeks.

* Is a walking caliper of any value?

No.

Operative Treatment for Fractures of the Shaft of the Femur

Give five indications for operative treatment using an intramedullary nail.

1. When interposed muscle mass prevents satisfactory closed reduction.
2. In middle aged or older people who would not tolerate twelve weeks in bed on traction.
3. Where there are other bones injured requiring treatment, intramedullary nailing can facilitate the management of other injuries.
4. Pathological fractures.
5. For economic reasons where there is a shortage of beds, the surgeon might lean towards internal fixation to enable the patient to go home in a week or ten days.

What is the best treatment for transverse fractures in the upper 1/3?

Kuntscher nail fixation.

What is meant by the closed technique of intramedullary nailing?

The nail is inserted in such a way that the fracture itself is not exposed.

When performing the closed intramedullary nailing technique, how is the fracture secured and maintained in the correct position?

By means of a Steinmann pin through the tibial tubercle, to which is attached weights to apply traction.

What is the name of the piece of metal that is passed through the greater trochanter down the shaft of the femur in the first stage of a blind nailing?

A guide wire.

When the two ends of the bone have been approximated under image intensifier X-ray control, what is the next step?

Push the guide wire down into the distal fragment.

How is the medullary cavity enlarged to take the nail?

A power operated cannulated reamer is passed over the correctly placed guide wire and the diameter of the medullary cavity is reamed to 12-16 mm.

What is the final stage of this closed method?

A nail of correct length and diameter is then passed over the guide wire and hammered down the shaft of the femur towards the knee.

When closed nailing is not possible, how would you proceed?

By open method in which the fracture is exposed through a lateral incision.

What is the next step after exposing the fracture?

The proximal and distal ends of the femur are reamed to the desired diameter and the nail may then be inserted from fracture site to greater trochanter or from greater trochanter to fracture site.

When the two ends of the femur are in the correct alignment with the medullary cavities opposite each other, what would you do?

The nail is driven home from above into the lower fragment.

After intramedullary nailing is it necessary to immobilize the patient in a splint or plaster?

No.

When might the patient start partial weight bearing?

Two weeks after the operation.

Treatment of Femoral Shaft Fractures in Children

For children under the age of four years, there is a special method. What is it?

Traction is applied by the gallows or Bryant traction device.

With these two methods, how is the traction attached to the limb?

By adhesive skin strapping applied direct to the child's lower limbs.

With gallows or Bryant traction, what weight would be applied to the traction device that stretches from the limbs to the overhead beams?

The traction should be sufficient to just lift the buttocks off the bed.

Since fractures of the femur unite rapidly in children under four, for how long would you retain the gallows or Bryant's traction?

About four weeks.

With regard to the traction on children's legs used for gallow's traction, why should the knees be kept slightly flexed by packed splints?

Occasionally keeping the knees extended leads to spasm of a major artery with ischaemia developing in the limbs.

What might be a complication of excessive and tight bandaging of the strapping to the limbs?

Again constriction of the blood vessels with ischaemia may occur.

What other precaution would you take to avoid this complication?

During the first four or five days, a constant watch should be made of the peripheral circulation in children in gallow's or Bryant's traction.

Complications of Fractures of the Shaft of the Femur

Three of these seven complications are common to all fractures. Give them first and then give the complete seven.

1. Delayed union.
2. Non-union.
3. Malunion.
4. Infection.
5. Injury to a major artery.
6. Injury to nerve.
7. Stiffness of the knee.

Delayed Union

When would you consider making the diagnosis of delayed union?

If unprotected weight bearing is not possible, after five months.

In the case of delayed union, is there any place for a full length plaster hip spica and allowing the patient to walk?

Yes, sometimes in younger people this method can stimulate further callus formation.

Non-union

What is the treatment here?

Bone grafting.

Give two techniques for bone grafting non-union of femur.

1. Kuntscher nail plus slivers of cancellous bone packed in the fracture site.
2. Plating of femur with cancellous bone placed at the fracture site.

Malunion

Malunion is rare but what is the commonest type of malunion?

Overlap with consequent shortening.

Give another common type of malunion.

Outward bowing in the upper third of the femur.

What long term effect might angular deformity have at the knee joint?

Osteoarthritis of the knee may be a sequel.

Treatment of Malunion

How would you treat shortening, say under 2 cm?

By a build up to the shoe.

If the malunion was of a very severe degree, would you consider refracturing the bone and realigning the fragments and holding with a plate or intramedullary nail?

Yes.

Is this common or rare?

Fairly common.

Infection

In the case of a compound fracture from without, would you recommend closing the skin after debridement or leaving it open?

With wounds that are heavily contaminated, it is best to leave them open and clean thoroughly and undertake delayed suture a few days later.

Injury to Major Artery

Is this common or rare?

It is rare.

Whose aid would you enlist for this problem?

That of a vascular surgeon.

Injury to Nerve

Which never is the commonest injured?

Sciatic nerve.

Stiffness of the Knee

Give two reasons for knee stiffness following fractured shaft of femur.

1. Adhesions between the muscle groups of the quadriceps inhibiting free gliding.
2. Adhesions between the muscles of the thigh and the fracture prevent full flexion of the knee.

Treatment of Knee Stiffness

How would you prevent this?

Continuation with active exercises is felt to be better than passively stretching the muscles about the knee.

Name one operation that might be used where quadriceps adhesion formation is very dense and prevents even slight knee movement.

Quadricepsplasty.

In essence, what is quadricepsplasty?

Division of all adhesions between the four muscles that constitute the quadriceps and the femur.

CHAPTER 17

DISLOCATION OF THE HIP

* Give the three types of traumatic dislocation of the hip — congenital dislocation of the hip is considered elsewhere.

1. Posterior dislocation or fracture dislocation.
2. Anterior dislocation.
3. Central fracture-dislocation.

* Which is the commonest of the three types of fracture-dislocation of the hip?

Posterior dislocation.

* What is the mechanics of a posterior dislocation?

A force applied along the long axis of the shaft of the femur with the hip flexed drives the femoral head out the back of the acetabulum.

* Give an example of this injury taking place.

Person sitting in front seat of a car in head-on collision and knee strikes heavily against dashboard with the hip and knee both flexed to about ninety degrees.

* In what percentage of cases of posterior dislocation is the acetabulum fractured?

Fifty percent.

* Where is the sciatic nerve in relation to the posterior dislocating head of femur?

It is directly in the line of displacement.

In which direction is the shaft of the femur rotated in a posterior dislocation?

Internally.

* How is the dislocation confirmed?

By X-ray which will also show a fracture in the acetabulum in fifty percent of cases.

* How would you conclude the sciatic nerve was injured?

By testing its motor, sensory and reflex function.

* In treatment of posterior dislocation of the hip, under a general anaesthetic the thigh is pulled in what direction?

Longitudinally.

* In what position is the hip joint held during the longitudinal pull?

The hip joint is flexed to a right angle.

* Since the deformity has internally rotated the shaft of the femur, how should the manipulator correct this?

By rotating the shaft of the femur externally or laterally.

* In the process of reducing the posterior dislocation, how is counter traction applied?

With the patient placed supine an assistant leans on the pelvis at the level of the iliac crests.

* How is the limb supported after reduction has been seen to be achieved clinically and radiologically?

Six weeks traction (Hamilton-Russell).

* If after reduction a large acetabular fragment is seen to be still unreduced, what would you do?

Open reduction must be carried out and the fragment replaced in the correct position and screwed there.

Complications

* Name four complications of posterior dislocation of the hip.

1. Injury to the sciatic nerve.
2. Post traumatic ossification.
3. Avascular necrosis of the femoral head.
4. Osteoarthritis.

* How is injury to the sciatic nerve treated initially?

By speedy reduction of the dislocation to relieve pressure on the nerve.

* What is the outlook with sciatic nerve injury in these cases?

If it is a neuro-praxia, the outlook is good. More severe damage to the sciatic nerve carries a poor prognosis.

* Why is there a poor prognosis with a severely damaged sciatic nerve at this point?

Because of the length of the nerve to be regenerated and because the distal muscles will have suffered irreversible changes before they are reinnervated.

Post traumatic ossification (see myositis ossificans).

* What percentage of heads of femur undergo avascular necrosis following posterior dislocation?

Fifteen-twenty percent.

How is it diagnosed?

Radiographs show increased density of head six weeks or more post accident.

* Does speed of reduction of the dislocation play a part in avascular necrosis?

Yes, the sooner the dislocation is reduced, the less likely is avascular necrosis to occur.

Why does avascular necrosis take place with posterior dislocation of the head of the femur?

1. Disruption of capsular vessels that supply the head.
2. Disruption of blood vessels in the ligamentum teres giving rise to reduction in blood flow to the head.

* How is avascular necrosis treated?

See management of osteoarthritis of hip.
Total hip replacement is often the treatment of choice for avascular necrosis.

* Osteoarthritis following posterior dislocation of femoral head. Give two reasons for this.

1. Secondary to avascular necrosis.
2. Roughening of the acetabulum from a fracture involving articular surface.

Which type of osteoarthritis develops the more quickly?

The osteoarthritis following avascular necrosis takes place more rapidly than the slower osteoarthritis seen when the acetabulum is disrupted.

* Give the two common ways of treating osteoarthritis nowadays.

1. Replacement arthroplasty, e.g. Charnley operation.
2. Arthrodesis of the hip joint (in the younger group).

Anterior Dislocation

* Is this common or rare?

Rare.

* What forces produce it? Give two.

1. Violent abduction force.
2. Violent lateral rotation force.

* Clinically what does the limb look like?

It is seen to be laterally rotated.

* How is it treated?

Reduce as early as possible then rest in traction as with posterior dislocation.

* Give two complications.

1. Osteoarthritis.
2. Avascular necrosis.

Central Fracture Dislocation

* In this condition what happens to the femoral head?

It is driven through the floor of the acetabulum into the pelvic cavity.

* Is the acetabulum always fractured?

Yes.

* How is the fracture dislocation sustained? Give two methods.

1. By a fall from a height onto the lateral aspect of the upper femur.
2. By a direct blow transmitted along the shaft of the femur with the hip joint abducted, e.g. motor vehicle accident — upper shin hitting dashboard.

* What range of acetabulum displacement might you see?

1. Just a few millimetres of inward displacement of the acetabulum.
2. The head might be driven right through the acetabulum into the pelvis.

* What is the main complication of this injury?

Subsequent osteoarthritis of the hip joint.

* Upon what factor does the development of osteoarthritis depend?

If the weight bearing part of the acetabulum is severely comminuted, then osteoarthritis in later life is almost certain. If, however, the weight bearing part of the acetabulum is in one piece and not comminuted, then osteoarthritic change may not take place.

In the treatment of this central dislocation of femur, how is the traction applied?

1. Through a Steinmann pin or screw passed through the greater trochanter.
2. Or by a green screw up the neck of the femur.

In which direction is the Steinmann pin passed?

Antero-posteriorly.

In which direction is traction applied?

Downwards and outwards, i.e. in the line of the neck of the femur.

As traction is applied to the femur in this way, in what percentage of cases does the acetabular fragment follow the head?

In the majority of cases, the acetabulum will be reduced into the correct position.

What would you do if a large piece of fractured acetabulum is still displaced?

Through an intrapelvic approach, the acetabular fragment should be screwed or wired back into the correct position.

After the central dislocation has been reduced, for how long would you continue to apply the traction?

Four-six weeks.

Is it more common or less common to have severe comminution of the acetabulum in this condition?

It is, unfortunately, more common to have severe comminution thus giving rise to osteo-arthritis in later life.

In this situation of severe comminution of acetabulum, is it possible to obtain a smooth articular surface?

No.

In cases of severe comminution, do some surgeons recommend leaving the head partially in the acetabulum and encouraging active mobilization after a two or three week rest in bed?

Yes.

What then, is the main complication of central dislocation of the hip?

Osteoarthritis.

What two operations might be of value to relieve the symptoms?

1. Total hip replacement.
2. Arthrodesis.

In the younger age group, say forty years of age or younger, would you recommend arthrodesis or total replacement arthroplasty?

Arthrodesis.

Why?

Because a successful arthrodesis is more permanent than replacement arthroplasty that may require revision if the cement or prostheses loosen after ten years or so.

CHAPTER 18

SUPRACONDYLAR FRACTURE OF THE FEMUR

In what direction is the fracture line in most supracondylar fractures?

Transverse immediately above the condyles.

In what direction might the fracture line extend?

Vertically down into the knee joint between the two femoral condyles.

What is the standard method of treating supracondylar fractures of the femur?

Thomas splint immobilization with a flexion knee piece and traction very similar to that used for a femoral shaft fracture.

How is traction attached?

Through Steinmann Pin in tibial tubercle or distal femur.

In these fractures, why is the degree of knee flexion important?

Because the amount of flexion can alter the position of the distal fragment.

What weight of traction is recommended?

About 9 kg.

What muscle pull tends to tilt the distal fragment backward?

The Gastrocnemius muscle.

How is this tilting corrected?

By further flexing the knee in the flexion knee piece, or padding under distal fragment thus creating a fulcrum.

When would you recommend the beginning of knee exercises in a supracondylar fracture being treated with this method?

Four weeks after the fracture was sustained.

Give an alternative method of treatment suitable for children with a supracondylar fracture.

Immobilization in a plaster hip spica. This enables the patient to get up and about non-weight bearing on crutches.

How might these fractures be internally fixated?

With a right angled blade plate.

Where is the blade situated?

Transversely through the condyles but distal to the fracture.

Where is the plate situated?

On the outer aspect of the shaft of the femur extending proximally across the fracture site.

How is the plate held to the femur?

With screws.

Give three indications for internally fixating these supracondylar fractures.

1. When conservative means have failed to reduce or hold the fracture adequately.
2. In elderly patients in order to mobilize them more speedily.
3. Occasionally younger patients for the same reason.

Complications of Supracondylar Fractures

Give the commonest complication.

Stiffness of the knee.

Give three less common complications.

1. Injury to the popliteal artery.
2. Injury to the major nerve trunk.
3. In children, growth plate disturbance.

Fractures of the Femoral Condyles

How are these produced?

By a direct blow.

Give two types of condylar fractures.

1. A crack.
2. Complete separation.

How would you treat an undisplaced crack?

In a long leg plaster of paris for eight weeks.

Why must displaced fractures be accurately reduced? Give two reasons.

1. Because knee function depends on correctly placed condyles.
2. To avoid osteoarthritis.

Give the conservative method for treating displaced condylar fractures.

Reduce the fracture under general anaesthesia and if position is good, then support limb in Thomas' splint for eight weeks (in continuous traction).

When would you operate?

If the above fails to secure perfect reduction.

At surgery, how would you hold the fracture?

By a long bolt or screw.

Give four complications of this fracture.

1. Stiff knee.
2. Osteoarthritis.
3. Injury to the artery.
4. Injury to the nerve.

CHAPTER 19

FRACTURES AND DISLOCATIONS OF THE PATELLA

* Give two mechanisms of fractures of the patella.

1. Violent contraction of quadriceps muscle as in stumbling.
2. A direct blow on the kneecap.

* Muscle pull gives rise to what type of fracture?

Usually a clean transverse fracture.

* A direct blow on the kneecap gives rise to what type of fracture?

Usually a comminuted stellate type of fracture.

Name a condition that can simulate a fracture of the patella radiologically.

A congenital bipartite patella may be confused with a fracture of patella.

In the normal patella radiologically, how many ossific centres are there?

One.

With bipartite patella, how many ossific or bony centres are there?

Two.

In bipartite patella, of the two pieces of bone where is the smaller usually found?

In the supero-lateral corner.

This smaller part of the patella appears to be ..... .

Separate.

Give four distinguishing features between a fracture of the patella and congenital bipartite patella.

1. In bipartite patella, the defect is nowhere near as tender as it would be with a fracture.
2. The margins of the gap in bipartite are smooth.
3. The site of the gap — supero-lateral corner — is uncommon for a fracture.
4. Radiographs of the other knee may well show the same congenital abnormality.

Treatment of Fractures of the Patella

* How would you treat a crack fracture?

1. Aspirate the blood from the knee joint.
2. Apply a plaster cylinder from groin to above ankle in about 5 degrees of flexion.

* For how long is the plaster worn?

Three weeks.

* What treatment would you recommend after plaster removal?

Active exercises.

* In cases of undisplaced cracked fracture of the patella, what holds the bony fragments together?

The aponeurosis.

* With regard to fracture of the patella with separation of the two fragments, is surgery necessary?

Yes, it is essential.

* Give two possible operations for a clean break with separation of the fragments.

1. Wiring the two fragments of the patella accurately together so the posterior surface is smooth or by screw fixation.
2. Excision of the patella.

* In a patient under forty, which operation would you recommend?

Screw fixation or wiring.

* In patients over forty, which operation would you recommend?

Some surgeons would recommend excision of the patella.

* After internal fixation of a fractured patella, for how long is plaster immobilization necessary?

Three weeks.

* After excision of the patella and suturing of the aponeurosis, for how long would you immobilize the limb in plaster?

Three weeks.

* After surgical treatment of a fractured patella, what follow up treatment would you recommend?

Physiotherapy to gradually restore full flexion and extension to the knee and build up the quadriceps muscles.

* If the posterior surface of the patella is left in an irregular roughened state, what complication ensues?

Osteoarthritis.

Comminuted Fracture of the Patella

* How would you treat this?

By excision of the patella in order to avoid osteoarthritis later in life.

Lateral Dislocation of the Patella

Name three types of lateral dislocation of the patella.

1. Acute dislocation. A solitary event.
2. Recurrent dislocation.
3. Habitual dislocation.

With recurrent dislocation and habitual dislocation, is there an abnormality in the patella?

Yes.

Acute Dislocation of the Patella

As the patella is displaced laterally by a violent force, in what position is the knee?

Flexed or semi-flexed.

Clinically, can the patient straighten the knee?

No.

Where is the tenderness most marked in this acute dislocation of the kneecap?

Antero-medially at the site of rupture of the capsule.

Treatment

How is the dislocation reduced?

By applying medialward pressure upon the patella while straightening the knee.

For how long should crepe bandage immobilization be instituted following reduction?

Four weeks.

Recurrent Dislocation of Patella

Is this more common in girls or boys?

Girls.

At what age does it usually occur initially?

Adolescence.

With recurrent dislocation, the kneecap slides laterally in the process of straightening. Give four reasons for this.

1. A generalized laxity of the joints.
2. An underdeveloped lateral condyle.
3. A high lying patella.
4. Genu valgum (knock knees).

Treatment of Recurrent Dislocation

Name one operation that is successful in treating this condition.

The re-attachment of the insertion of the patella tendon to a point more medial to its original insertion, i.e. Hauser's operation.

Name a complication of Hauser's operation.

It may lead to patello-femoral osteoarthritis.

Give an alternative method and give its advantage and a disadvantage.

Excision of the patella thus making osteoarthritis at patello-femoral joint impossible. However tendon may dislocate.

What is meant by habitual dislocation?

Every time the knee is bent the patella dislocates.

What is the basic cause of habitual dislocation?

Shortening of the quadriceps muscle.

In particular, what muscle is shortened?

Vastus lateralis.

What other abnormality in vastus lateralis might be seen?

An abnormal fibrous band may join vastus lateralis to the ilio-tibial tract thus tending to pull the patella out of its groove.

How is habitual dislocation best treated?

By releasing the tight muscle or band sufficiently to allow a normal movement of the patella.

CHAPTER 20

FRACTURES OF THE TIBIAL PLATEAU

From above down, there are three groups of fractures of the tibia and fibula. What are they?

1. Fractures of the condyles of the tibia.
2. Fractures of the shafts of the tibia and fibula separately or together.
3. Fractures and fracture dislocations about the ankle.

Which of the condylar fractures is the commoner?

The lateral condyle.

See if you can deduce how the lateral tibial condyle would be fractured.

By a blow that abducts the tibia on the femur while the foot is fixed on the ground, e.g. bumper of car striking outer side of knee of pedestrian.

With this type of bumper fracture, which ligament would you expect to be stretched or ruptured?

The medial ligament of the knee.

Fracture of the Lateral Tibial Condyle

Name three types of fractures of the lateral tibial condyle.

1. Compression fracture with fragmentation — the commonest type.
2. Depressed plateau fracture without severe fragmentation.
3. Oblique shearing fracture.

The compression fracture with fragmentation is the commonest and is produced by crushing impact of the lateral ..... of ..... .

Condyle; Femur.

With the depressed plateau type, there is little fragmentation and a large part of the articular surface of the lateral condyle is ..... but remains as a single ..... .

Depressed.
Piece.

The oblique shearing fracture is also ..... and in this situation, there is an oblique ..... that has sheared off a large part of the ..... .

Rare.
Fracture.
Condyle.

Treatment of Tibial Condyle Fractures

The common compression fracture with fragmentation is best treated with rigid immobilization or active exercises. Which?

Active exercises.

In the early stage with these fractures, the patient is confined to ..... and any tense haemarthrosis is ..... .

Bed.
Aspirated.

A plaster slab is applied to protect the knee from unguarded movements at night time, but during the day the plaster splint is removed and ..... commenced.

Exercises.

When would you allow the patient out of bed to take partial weight?

Between the third and sixth week after the accident.

By the time the patient gets out of bed, full movements at the knee would have been restored.

Treatment of Depressed Plateau Fracture without Fragmentation

Is it possible in these fractures to restore the articular surface of the tibial condyle to something approaching normal?

Yes.

Through a window in the antero-lateral cortex of the tibia, a little below the level of the ....., the depressed fragment is ..... from below until its articular surface is flush with the surrounding cartilage.

Joint.
Elevated.

How would you know when the depressed fragment has been correctly replaced?

By direct viewing of the articular cartilage through an upward prolongation of the incision that opens the knee joint.

This procedure would leave a cavity in the lower part of the tibial condyle; how would you deal with this?

The cavity is filled with cancellous bone chips, or a triangular piece of bone graft.

Oblique Shearing Fractures of the Lateral Tibial Condyle

Give two ways of treating shearing fractures of tibial condyle.

1. Manipulation and reduction.
2. Operative reduction and internal fixation.

Manipulative reduction can be carried out with the aid of a few taps from a ..... .

Mallet.

How would you prevent the mallet from damaging the skin in your attempt to elevate the fractured condyle?

By tapping the skin after it had been covered with two turns of an esmarch rubber bandage.

Having reduced it closed, how would you prevent refracturing of the tibia?

By enclosing the limb in a full-length plaster of paris.

After ..... weeks' immobilization, start the ..... programme.

Four; Exercise.

If manipulation fails, the fracture is opened and repositioned and held with the aid of a large ..... or ....

Screw.
Buttress plate.

Complications of Fractures of the Lateral Tibial Condyle

Complications are readily calculated and number three. What are they?

1. Genu valgum.
2. Joint stiffness.
3. Late osteoarthritis.

Genu valgum — is this common or rare?

Common, but of minor degree.

Stiffness of the knee — how would one treat this?

With active physiotherapy.

Osteoarthritis — why does this develop?

Due to damage to articular cartilage.

Once osteoarthritis has developed, give three possible ways of treating it surgically.

1. Corrective osteotomy by removal of medial wedge from upper tibia.
2. Knee replacement operation.
3. Arthrodesis of knee. Very rare.

Fractures of the Medial Tibial Condyle

Since these fractures are a mirror image of fractures of the lateral condyle, its features and treatment are comparable to those of the lateral condylar fractures.

CHAPTER 21

LIGAMENTOUS INJURIES ABOUT THE KNEE

Tears of the Medial Ligament

What sort of force injures the medial ligament?

An abduction force.

Would you consider that the knee is momentarily subluxated?

Yes, but it returns to normal position immediately.

What ligaments would prevent a very wide abduction of the knee joint?

The cruciate ligaments together with the medial ligament would have to be ruptured for a wide abduction.

Clinically the joint is filled with ..... fluid.

Bloodstained.

Which end of the medial collateral ligament is torn?

Usually the upper femoral attachment of the medial ligament.

With regard to diagnosis, how do you tell if the rupture of the medial ligament is complete or partial?

Using antero-posterior radiographs, apply an abduction stress to the knee joint with the patient under general anaesthetic.

With complete rupture of the ligament, what do you see on the radiograph?

The joint opens up on the medial side.

If the joint opens very widely on the medial side, name three structures that would be ruptured.

1. The cruciate ligaments.
2. The capsule.
3. The medial ligament.

How would you treat a tear of the medial ligament that causes only slight opening up of the joint under general anaesthetic?

Conservative treatment with aspiration of blood and long leg plaster retained for six weeks.

How would you treat the condition if there was wide abduction of the knee with probable cruciate and capsule tear as well as medial ligament tear?

Exploration of the knee on the inner side should be undertaken.

What would you do if the meniscus is seen to be torn?

Remove it, or repair a peripheral tear.

What would you do if the cruciate ligament is seen to be torn?

Probably leave it alone unless repair to cruciate is practicable.

How would you treat the tear in the capsule?

Repair it.

How do you treat the laceration in the medial ligament itself?

Repair it.

How long do you immobilize the knee after this type of surgery?

Six weeks.

With both conservative and operative treatment, what would you suggest by way of physiotherapy after the plaster has been removed?

Intensive exercises and heat to restore full flexion and extension to the knee.

Tear of the Lateral Ligament

Is this more or less common than medial ligament tear?

Much less common.

What force produces it?

An adducting force to the tibia upon the femur.

This type of adduction force may produce what type of injury to the head of the fibula?

An avulsion fracture of the head of the fibula.

In view of what has been said immediately above, what nerve might be injured with this type of accident?

The lateral popliteal nerve might be injured (common peroneal).

How would you treat a tear of the lateral ligament?

Usually conservatively, i.e. four weeks in plaster of paris.

Tears of the Cruciate Ligament

The cruciate ligaments can be torn in conjunction with a rupture of the medial or lateral ligaments of the knee. How would an isolated tear, say of the anterior cruciate ligament, come to pass — what is the mechanism of this?
Give two.

1. The anterior ligament is torn by a force driving the tibia forwards relative to the femur.
2. Hyperextension of the knee may also tear it.

How is the posterior cruciate ligament torn?

By a force driving the upper end of the tibia backwards.

Give two methods of treatment of cruciate ligaments.

Some schools feel that the results of surgical treatment are so poor that conservative treatment in a plaster cylinder for three weeks should be followed by intensive physiotherapy to build up the quadriceps muscle.
Others feel, however, that re-constitution of the freshly injured cruciate ligament is well worthwhile.

Does a ruptured anterior cruciate ligament leave severe knee disability?

No, people play squash and tennis with this disability provided the quadriceps muscle is strong.

Avulsion of the Tibial Spine

How is avulsion of the tibial spine sustained?

In the same way as cruciate ligament injury.

Is the cruciate ligament itself intact?

Yes.

Give two ways of treating avulsion of the tibial spine.

Most cases — straighten the knee and put it in plaster for six weeks.   If bone fragment is still elevated from the tibia, it might have to be replaced and held in position with a screw, or wire.

Strain of Medial or Lateral Ligament

* Is this common or rare?

It is probably the commonest condition one sees in the knee.

* What force will strain the medial ligament?

An abduction force.

95

* What force will strain the lateral ligament?   An adduction force.

Clinical Features of Strain of Medial or Lateral Ligament

* What is the nature of the strain applied to the knee?   Abduction strain for medial ligament strain. Adduction strain for lateral ligament strain.

* Where might the tenderness be?   Either the upper or the lower attachment or in the mid section of the ligament.

* What makes the pain worse?   Stretching the appropriate ligament.

* What happens to the flexion and extension range of the knee?   Flexion is slightly restricted due to pain at the site of the injured ligament.

Diagnosis of a Medial or Lateral Ligament Strain

* With what condition might this be confused?   A tear of the medial meniscus.

* May the two injuries co-exist?   Yes.

* With strain, how long does the effusion in the knee last?   About two weeks.

* If, for example, the limitation of extension and effusion persists for more than say three weeks, one would think in terms of the injury being due to a ....   Torn meniscus.

* How long does the pain of a strained medial or lateral ligament last?   Up to ten weeks.

Treatment

* How would you immobilize the knee to rest the injured ligament?   In a cast.

* For how long would the immobilization last?   Two weeks.

* What would be the extent of the plaster or hexalite?   From groin to above malleoli.

Pelligrini-Steida's Disease

In this condition, as a result of a strain to the ligament, ossification occurs at what site?   At the upper attachment of the medial ligament of the knee.

What pathological change takes place in the initial injury?   Haematoma formation goes on to ossification or bone formation.

Clinically, there is a history of ..... to the medial ligament.   Injury.

What would one find on examining the knee?   Thickening and slight tenderness at the upper attachment of the medial collateral ligament (adjacent to the medial femoral condyle).

What is seen on the radiographs?   Bone formation or calcification adjacent to medial femoral condyle.

How would you treat Pelligrini-Steida's disease?   By active mobilizing exercises and a muscle strengthening programme.

CHAPTER 22

MENISCAL TEARS

* What is the other name for the meniscus?

Semi-lunar cartilage.

* How many cartilages are there?

Two in each knee.

* Where are they located?

Between the femoral condyle proximally and the tibial plateau distally.

* What shape are they?

C shape.

* What are they called?

The medial meniscus and the lateral meniscus.

* Tears of the menisci cause internal ..... of the knee.

Derangement.

* In which sex is this injury more common?

Male.

* How is the tear produced?

By a twisting force with the knee semi-flexed or fully flexed and weight bearing. Then as the slightly abducted knee is straightened, the femoral condyle splits the meniscus from front to back.

* In which sport does it commonly occur?

Football, i.e. soccer or rugby.

* In what labouring work is it common due to the squatting position?

In coal mining.

* Which is the most common meniscus to be torn?

The medial meniscus.

Pathology of Tears of the Menisci

* Name three types of meniscal tears.

1. Bucket-handle tear.
2. Anterior horn tear.
3. Posterior horn tear.

* In the common bucket-handle tear, there is a longitudinal split that extends through the length of the ..... and in this bucket-handle tear, the fragments remain ..... at both ends.

Meniscus.
Attached.

* Which is the commonest type of injury?

Bucket-handle tear.

* Which is the bucket-handle?

The central fragment that is displaced towards the middle of the joint.

* In this situation, the condyle of the femur rolls upon the tibia through the rent in the ..... .

Meniscus.

* The classical symptom of the bucket-handle tear is that it limits full ..... and this lack of full extension is called ..... .

Extension.
Locking.

* The femoral condyle is so shaped that it requires most space when the knee is ..... .

Straight.

* So the chief effect of a displaced bucket-handle fragment is that it limits full ..... .

Extension.

If the initial longitudinal tear emerges at the concave border of the meniscus, a ..... tag is formed.

Pedunculated.

In two situations, the pedunculated tag remains attached to the anterior or posterior horn, thus a posterior horn tear remains attached to the posterior horn and the anterior horn tear remains attached to the ..... horn.

Anterior.

What significance do you attach to the transverse tear through the meniscus?

It is always an artefact produced at the time of operation.

Since the menisci are avascular, why is the knee sometimes filled with blood at the time of surgery?

The blood is due to an associated tearing of the synovia.

Do torn menisci heal spontaneously?

No.

Clinical Features of Torn Menisci

* What is the common age group for torn menisci?

Eighteen — forty five years.

* What is the usual history given?

A twisting injury to the flexed knee whilst taking weight, associated with severe pain on the inner side of the knee.

* Where is the pain usually located?

Along the medial joint line.

* When the patient attempts to straighten the knee, he finds he is ..... to.

Unable.

* This phenomenon is known as ..... .

Locking.

* As a result of synovial irritation, the knee then ..... .

Swells.

* Sometimes the knee settles down and it can be straightened, i.e. it unlocks. Two or three weeks later with a slight twisting strain, again the knee ..... .

Locks.

* The main symptoms then of a torn medial meniscus are five in number. What are they?

1. Pain on the inner side of the knee.
2. Effusion.
3. Locking.
4. Clicking.
5. Giving way.

* By locking, one means limitation of ..... .

Extension.

This phenomenon is not always appreciated by the patient who simply feels the knee won't straighten completely.

* It is thought that true locking in which the knee simply won't fully extend the last few degrees is caused only by a .... tear.

Bucket-handle.

* Tag tears cause momentary ..... of the knee, but not true locking.

Catching.

* Physical examination is carried out in the usual way by observing the knee under the following headings. What are they?

1. Inspection.
2. Palpation.
3. Movement.
4. X-ray.

What might be seen on looking at the knee that houses a torn cartilage?

1. Swelling or effusion.
2. Wasting of quadriceps muscle.
3. The knee is held slightly flexed.

On feeling, we find that there is ..... along the ..... joint line.

Tenderness.
Antero-medial.

* Also on feeling, we can see that the last few degrees have a springy resistance when one attempts to straighten the knee fully.

* The attempt to fully straighten the knee produces ..... .

Pain.

Measurement of the quadriceps muscle confirms ..... of that muscle.

Wasting.

* What is the McMurray's sign?

Passive rotation of the tibia on the femur with the knee flexed and an abducting force applied gives rise to a painful click at site of the injured cartilage as the knee is gradually extended.

* The radiographs usually show ..... .

Nothing.

* What is the main clinical difference between a tear of the medial meniscus and a tear of the lateral meniscus?

Usually with the lateral meniscus, the pain is on the lateral joint line, rather than on the medial.

* As an aid to diagnosis, the most modern methods of investigating a knee are with the aid of an ..... and ..... .

Arthroscope; Arthrogram.

* Generally speaking if there is any doubt as to whether or not the cartilage is torn, one acts conservatively and gives physiotherapy to build up the quadriceps as in this way, the attacks might settle down for many years.

* What do you think might happen with a knee that has a torn cartilage that is causing repeated locking episodes over a long period of time?

Osteoarthritis might develop.

* When it comes to surgical treatment, this takes the form of excision of part or whole of the meniscus — which?

The whole meniscus.

* Some surgeons prefer to remove the .... fragment alone.

Bucket-handle.

* Finally, unlocking of the locked knee may be achieved by ..... under anaesthesia and this sometimes completes the tear of the bucket-handle enabling the knee to straighten fully and displacing the bucket-handle part into the intercondylar region.

Manipulation.

* The patient is thus made more ..... whilst awaiting surgery.

Comfortable.

CHAPTER 23

FRACTURES OF THE SHAFTS OF THE TIBIA AND THE FIBULA

* There are two types of force that will fracture the shafts of the tibia and fibula. What are they?

1. An angulatory force.
2. A rotational force.

* Which force do you think would cause a transverse fracture?

An angulatory force.

* Fractures resulting from a rotational force are usually ..... .

Spiral.

* With rotational force fractures of tibia and fibula, are the fractures at the same or at different levels in the two bones?

Different levels.

* With fractures of an angulatory force, the fractures of tibia and fibula are usually at the ..... level.

Same.

* What is the commonest cause of fractures of the shafts of the tibia and fibula?

Motor cycle accidents.

Treatment of Fractures of the Shafts of the Tibia and Fibula

* With fractures of tibia and fibula, the fibula fracture can usually be ..... .

Disregarded.

* The reason for it being disregarded is that it plays little part in ..... bearing and it nearly always ..... readily.

Weight.
Unites.

* With fractures of the tibia, ... should still be the method of choice.

Conservative treatment.

* With the leg in a long-leg plaster, the patient can get about on a pair of ..... .

Crutches.

* The accepted method of treatment is to reduce the fracture by manipulation and to ..... the limb in a full length plaster cast.

Immobilize.

* At what angle should the knee be held in the long plaster cast?

Very slightly flexed.

* How high does the plaster extend with fractures of the tibia and fibula?

To the groin.

* How far down does the cast reach?

To the metatarsal heads.

* At what angle is the ankle held?

At a right angle.

* What is meant by wedging the plaster cast?

By dividing the plaster cast two-thirds of the way around its circumference at the level of the fracture, angulation of the fracture can be corrected by wedging the plaster open at the appropriate point.

* If the fracture is transverse, ... should be encouraged after two or three weeks. — Walking.

* In order to facilitate walking, a ..... or ..... is applied to the under-surface of the cast. — Heel; Rocker.

* If the fracture is oblique and, therefore, unstable, walking on the affected leg should be ..... for about six weeks. — Deferred.

* How long does a fractured tibia usually take to unite? — Between three and four months.

* When the fracture has united, how does one regain movement in the knee and ankle? — With supervised physiotherapy.

What is meant by functional bracing? — Here, the full length cast is exchanged after a week or so for one that liberates knee and ankle.

Operative Treatment for Fractures of the Tibia and Fibula

* Give two indications for operative intervention with fractures of the tibia and fibula. — 1. When the fracture cannot be reduced adequately by manipulation. 2. When plaster of paris fails to maintain an acceptable position of the fragments.

* What is the commonest method of internal fixation of a fractured tibia? — A plate and screws.

How many screws are on either side of the fracture? — Three or four usually.

On which surface is the plate attached in a fractured tibia? — On the lateral surface rather than the subcutaneous surface.

Give three advantages of closed intramedullary Kuntscher nailing of the tibia. — 1. There is no scarring in front of the shin. 2. The chance of infection is greatly reduced. 3. It gives greater rigidity than plating and thus enables the patient to commence early weight-bearing.

What is meant by the "closed" technique of intramedullary nailing? — With this method, the fracture itself is not exposed.

Fractures of the Shaft of the Tibia Alone

* Is this a common or rare phenomenon? — Rare.

* Is the displacement less severe or more severe than when both bones are fractured? — Less severe due to the splinting effect of the intact fibula.

* With regard to treatment, in most cases the fragments can be held adequately by a .... plaster. — Full; Length.

* In what way may the intact fibula act as a disadvantage? — It may prevent the tibial surfaces from coming together in close apposition.

If the strut-like effect of the intact fibula is a hindrance, what can be done about it? — Excise a short length of the fibula.

Fatigue Fracture of Tibia

What is a fatigue fracture?

A fracture produced by repeated minor stresses rather than by a major injury.

Where else does one see fatigue fractures?

In metatarsal bones.

What is the other name for a fatigue fracture?

Stress fracture.

Give three unaccustomed activities that might produce a fatigue fracture of the tibia.

Walking, running or dancing.

Symptoms are that of ..... over the tibia.

Pain.

Physical examination shows local .... over the site of the fracture.

Tenderness.

What is seen on the radiograph of a stress fracture?

A faint transverse crack.

How is a fatigue fracture of the tibia treated?

A few weeks in a full length plaster is advised.

Congenital Pseudarthrosis of Tibia in Childhood

In which half of the tibia is this likely to be seen?

In the lower half.

Is pseudarthrosis of the tibia congenital or acquired?

Congenital. It is a congenital abnormality.

Are these fractures easy to treat with conservative treatment or with bone grafting?

No, they are resistant to both conservative treatment and bone grafting.

Fractures generally in children heal very quickly and readily but this is not the case with ....

Congenital pseudarthrosis.

In many cases, pseudarthrosis of the tibia is associated with another condition. What is it?

Neurofibromatosis.

If the fracture cannot be made to heal, what happens to limb length?

It is seriously impaired.

The ultimate treatment for this condition is .....

Amputation.

What is the best way of treating pseudarthrosis of the tibia in childhood?

Intramedullary nailing giving rigid fixation plus cancellous bone grafting and electrical stimulation.

This method usually succeeds but as the limb grows, something might have to be done about the Kuntscher nail. What is it?

Repeated operations may be required for the insertion of larger nails as the limb grows.

Fracture of the Fibula Alone

Are these fractures common or rare?

Rare.

Fractures of the fibula alone are produced by a direct ..... over the bone.

Blow.

Does this fracture interfere with walking?

No. Therefore the fracture may be overlooked.

How are these fractures best treated?

A below-knee walking plaster for three weeks is usually sufficient.

In fact, a fracture of the shaft of the fibula is the constant accompaniment of rupture of the inferior ..... ligament.

Tibiofibular.

Separation then of the lower end of the tibia from the lower end of the fibula is called ..... diastasis.

Tibiofibular.

Fatigue Fracture of the Fibula

What is the other name for fatigue fracture?

Stress fracture.

In what part of the fibula do we commonly see fatigue fracture?

In the lowest third.

May they also occur in the middle or uppermost third?

Yes.

With fatigue fracture of the fibula, is there a history of sudden injury?

No.

Name two activities that might cause this type of stress fracture.

An unusual amount of walking or running.

What does one see in the early radiographs of a fatigue fracture of the fibula?

A faint hairline crack.

What does one see on the later radiographs of a stress fracture of the fibula?

The fracture is made evident by surrounding callus.

Complications of Fractures of Tibia and Fibula

* Name three complications that can occur with almost any fracture.

1. Delayed union.
2. Non-union.
3. Malunion.

* Name two additional complications that are seen with fractures of the tibia.

1. Infection going on to osteomyelitis.
2. Damage to an important artery or nerve.

Why are fractures of the tibia so often associated with osteomyelitis?

Because the tibia is only covered by skin anteriorly and therefore, a breach of the skin gives easy access for germs into the bone.

Infection of Fractures of the Tibia and Fibula

Give three reasons why infection as a complication of compound fractures of the tibia is less common now than it used to be.

1. Contamination is reduced by prompt cleansing of the wound, i.e. debridement.
2. By use of local antibiotics.
3. By the use of general systemic antibiotics.

Give two signs that would make one suspect the fracture is infected.

1. There would be a suppurative odour from the plaster.
2. A persistent pyrexia.

In that event, the ..... must be split and free drainage provided by opening up the ..... .

Plaster.
Wound.

At a later date, fragments of dead bone known as ..... may have to be removed.

Sequestra.

When the infection has been overcome, healing may be hastened by applying .... grafts to the granulating surface of the skin.

Split-skin.

What is the major complication if serious infection takes place at the fracture site?

Union is delayed or prevented.

Delayed Union and Non-union

If the union has not been established by the sixteenth week, what type of operation is recommended if the skin be healthy?

Bone grafting.

Give two methods of bone grafting suitable for the tibia.

1. A sliding bone graft from the same tibia is screwed to the lateral surface of the bone.
2. A phemister graft using slivers of cancellous bone from the iliac crest are inserted beneath the periosteum and the fracture itself is not disturbed.

What type of internal fixation might be used in conjunction with the phemister graft?

Intramedullary nailing.

What might you have to do if the fibula is obstructing the apposition of the ends of the tibia?

The fibula in this case might be divided, i.e. osteotomised.

In many cases of delayed union of the tibia, the fibular fracture is soundly ..... .

United.

If there has been some absorption at the tibial fracture site, a united fibula might actually hold the tibial fragments ..... .

Apart.

In this event, consideration should be given to excising a small length of ..... .

Fibula.

This quite simple manoeuvre can frequently lead to ..... of the un-united tibial fracture.

Union.

Damage to Artery or Nerve

Fractures of the upper end of the tibia are liable to injure which artery?

Popliteal artery.

What else might injure the popliteal artery apart from a fragment of tibia?

A plaster cast or dressing that is too tight.

Which nerve is likely to be damaged with a fractured tibia?

The lateral popliteal nerve (common peroneal).

In what part of the limb would one expect to see signs of impaired circulation?

Since the patient is usually in a plaster cast, the toes must be observed for colour, temperature and feeling-sensation.

What would you do if, on examination, the toes are found to be cold, blue and numb?

Instantly split the plaster and underlying padding and open it up till colour and feeling returns and then re-apply a new cast which is less constricting.

Malunion

What are the two common types of malunion?

1. Shortening.
2. Angulation at the fracture site.

Angulation at the fracture site, if it be a fracture of the upper tibia, can give rise to what problems with the knee at a later date?

Osteoarthritis of the knee.

How would you correct a large angular deformity of a united fracture of the tibia?

Osteotomy and straightening of the bent bone might help.

FOR POST-GRADUATE STUDENTS ONLY

Technique of Intramedullary Nailing for Tibial Fractures

The operation may be carried out by the ..... technique without ..... the fracture.

Closed.
Exposing.

How may the reduction be aided in those cases that are to be nailed by the closed technique?

By Steinmann pin in the lower tibia, or calcaneus.

With the blind or closed technique, at what angle is the knee held flexed?

At 120 degrees of flexion.

With the closed technique where is the incision made?

Medial to the patellar tendon to expose the intercondylar ridge.

A guide wire is introduced near the front of this ..... ridge and pushed down the medullary canal as far as the ..... .

Intercondylar.
Fracture.

How is the medullary cavity increased to the appropriate size for the intramedullary nail?

By means of a cannulated reamer that passes over the correctly placed guide wire.

When the medullary canal has been reamed up to about ..... millimetres in diameter, a nail of appropriate size is hammered over the guide into the proximal and then ..... fragments.

Twelve.

Distal.

Following intramedullary fixation, is a plaster necessary?

No.

When is weight-bearing permitted after intramedullary nailing?

Two or three weeks post-operation.

Does the intercondylar ridge of the tibia play any part in the articular surface on the knee joint?

No, therefore the nail can be passed through the intercondylar ridge with impunity.

End of Technique of Intramedullary Nailing for Tibial Fractures

Operative Treatment for Fractures of the Tibia and Fibula (Cont'd.)

Give five other methods of internally fixing fractures of the tibia.

1. Transfixion screws.
2. Circumferential wires.
3. Metal plates and screws.
4. Cortical bone grafts, held by screws.
5. External fixateur.

In what type of fracture would you use transfixion screws?

Oblique or spiral fractures.

Does one need to use a plaster cast as well as one or two screws?

Yes.

When would one use circumferential wires?

In long oblique fractures as an alternative to transfixion screws.

When a metal plate and screws are used, on what surface should the plate be attached?

On the submuscular surface. It should never be placed on the subcutaneous surface.

Give one further method of immobilizing a fractured tibia.

By a sliding bone graft.

In this situation, whence is the bone graft derived?

From the same tibia.

What additional advantage does it have over a metal plate?

It probably promotes union of the fracture.

In the case of a fractured tibia that has extensive blistering on the skin or soft tissue wounding, how else may this be treated?

By continuous weight traction with limb in a plaster back slab or resting in a Thomas' splint or Bohler Frame.

Where is the pin situated for the application of traction?

In the tibia — never in the calcaneum because of pin tract infection.

How long would one keep the traction on before immobilizing the patient in a closed plaster cylinder?

About four weeks.

External fixation may be achieved by using dual ..... pins above and ..... the fracture. In this method, the ends of the pins are incorporated in a ..... or in a special adjustable ..... device.

Transfixion; Below.

Plaster; Fixation.

CHAPTER 24

FRACTURES AND FRACTURE DISLOCATIONS ABOUT THE ANKLE

With regards to frequency of injury, where do the bones of the ankle joint rate compared to fractures of the lower end of the radius?

Bones of the ankle joint are the second most commonly injured after fractures of the lower end of the radius.

Sometimes fractures about the ankle joint are grouped together under the general title of ..... fractures.

Potts.

Mechanism of Injury and Patterns of Fracture

* There are three types of injury depending upon the forces causing them. What are the three types of injury?

1. Abduction plus or minus lateral rotation force (the commonest type).
2. Adduction force.
3. Vertical compression force.

* The above indicates the mechanism of the injury and the fracture or fracture-dislocations are divided into ..... distinct groups.

Eight.

* What are the eight distinct groups of fracture or fracture-dislocation about the ankle joint?

1. Isolated fracture of lateral malleolus.
2. Isolated fracture of medial malleolus.
3. Fracture of the lateral malleolus with lateral shift of the talus.
4. Fracture of both malleoli with displacement of the talus.
5. Tibiofibular diastasis.
6. Posterior marginal fracture of the tibia with posterior displacement of the talus.
7. Vertical compression fracture of the lower articular surface of the tibia.
8. Epiphyseal plate fractures.

General Principles of Treatment

* How would one treat fractures without displacement?

Generally speaking, a below knee walking plaster for three to six weeks is adequate.

* In fractures with displacement, the talus has to be restored to its normal relationship with the tibiofibular mortise. In addition, the tibia and the fibula must be in normal relationship one to the other.

* Reduction is affected by ..... under ..... .

Manipulation; Anaesthetic.

* In what direction are the malleolar fragments manipulated in order to affect a reduction?

These bones must be manipulated in a direction **opposite** to the direction of the displacement.

* Having reduced the fracture, it is held in the correct position in a ....

Plaster of paris cast.

* For how long should this type of fracture be in plaster?

For eight to ten weeks.

* Since the fractures might slip in a plaster, check ..... should be obtained a week after reduction.

Radiographs.

* Supposing one is unable to get the fibula fragments and talus in the correct position, how would one secure the fractured bone?

By screw fixation.

* Following screw fixation, is plaster immobilization necessary?

In most cases, yes.

Complications of Ankle Fractures

* Name two.

1. Stiffness of the ankle.
2. Later, osteoarthritis.

Give three ways in which ankle stiffness might be prevented.

1. By active exercises.
2. By elevation of the crepe-bandaged limb when resting.
3. Internal fixation and early motion.

The enclosed diagram depicts 14 types of injuries, the names of which have been obliterated. Name each of the 14 types of injury, depicted in the diagrams on page 110.

1. Shearing fracture of lateral malleolus.
2. Avulsion fracture of the medial malleolus.
3. Fracture of lateral malleolus, rupture of medial ligament plus lateral shift of talus.
4. Fracture of lateral and medial malleoli plus lateral shift of talus.
5. Tibiofibula diastasis, rupture of the tibio-fibula and medial ligaments plus fracture of shaft of fibula and lateral shift of talus.
6. Posterior marginal fracture of tibial articular surface plus posterior shift of the talus with associated adduction fracture.
7. Strain of lateral ligament.
8. Shearing fracture of medial malleolus.
9. Avulsion fracture of lateral malleolus.
10. Complete rupture of lateral ligament.
11. Fracture of medial and lateral malleoli plus medial shift of talus.
12. Posterior marginal fracture of tibial articular surface plus posterior shift of talus with associated abduction fracture.
13. Anterior marginal fracture of tibia plus anterior shift of talus.
14. Comminuted fracture of tibial articular surface plus fracture of fibula plus an upward displacement of talus.

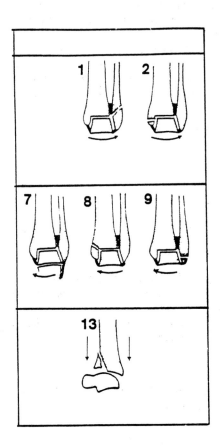

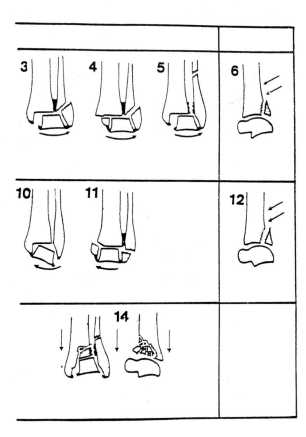

Reproduced from "Outline of Fractures"
by J. Crawford Adams
by kind permission of the author
and the publishers —
Churchill Livingstone — Edinburgh.

What factors predispose to osteoarthritis of the joint following fracture involving that joint? Give two factors.

1. If the fracture involves the articulating ankle surfaces causing roughness between the moving bones, this will predispose to osteoarthritis.
2. If the talus is left as a sloppy fit between the two malleoli due to inadequate reduction, this too will give rise to excessive wear and tear and later osteoarthritis might develop.

Give one operation that can be used to treat osteoarthritis in the ankle joint.

Arthrodesis.

Is it possible to do a joint replacement on the ankle?

Yes.

Isolated Fractures of the Lateral Malleolus

Of the fourteen recognized fractures of the ankle, which numbers are attached to those demonstrating an isolated fracture of the lateral malleolus?

Numbers 1 and 9.

Give three mechanisms whereby an isolated fracture of the lateral malleolus may be sustained.

1. It may be sheared off by an abduction force.
2. It may be sheared off by a lateral rotation force (the commonest).
3. Lateral malleolus may be avulsed by an adduction force.

With isolated fractures of the lateral malleolus, is there any displacement of the talus?

No.

Why is there no displacement of the talus?

Because the medial malleolus and the medial ligaments are intact.

Are the malleolar fragments in this group displaced usually?

No, usually not displaced.

Describe the fractures seen in figures 2, 6 and 8.

They are isolated fractures of a malleolus.

Treatment of Isolated Fractures of the Lateral Malleolus

Is union of these fractures a problem?

No, they almost all unite with immobilization.

Is plaster immobilization essential?

No, it is mainly to relieve pain.

In order to relieve pain then a below knee cast is applied for ..... weeks.

Three.

When the plaster has been removed, how is the ankle best treated?

With heat and exercises.

Isolated Fractures of the Medial Malleolus

Of the fourteen recognized fractures about the ankle, what numbers represent isolated fractures of the medial malleolus?

Numbers 2 and 8.

Give two mechanisms whereby this fracture might be sustained.

1. Shearing off of medial malleolus by adduction force.
2. Avulsion of medial malleolus by abduction force.

Where most isolated fractures of lateral malleolus heal readily, fractures of the medial malleolus have a complication that not only prevents reduction but also prevents union. What is that complication?

A fringe of periosteum may be turned in between the separated bone fragments causing reduction to be difficult and union to be hindered.

Treatment of Isolated Fractures of the Medial Malleolus

Most of these fractures are treated by closed or by open methods. Which?

Usually by open reduction.

How are these fractures held following open reduction?

By a long transfixing screw driven upwards from the tip of the malleolus.

Is plaster of paris used after the operation?

Yes.

What is the usual angle between the sole of the foot and the line of the tibia after plaster has been applied?

Ninety degrees.

For how long does the plaster remain?

Eight weeks.

When is walking permitted after internal screw fixation in these cases?

After two or three weeks.

If perfect apposition can be achieved without screw fixation, then simple below-knee plaster immobilization is instituted (after manipulation) for an .... period.

Eight week.

Fracture of the Lateral Malleolus with Lateral Displacement of the Talus

Which diagram represents this type of fracture?

Diagram 3.

What force would produce this type of fracture of lateral malleolus with lateral displacement of the talus?

An abduction or lateral rotation force.

Since the talus is shifted laterally and the medial malleolus is intact, which ligament must have ruptured for this event to take place?

The medial ligament.

What is the other name for the medial ligament?

Deltoid ligament.

How is the shift of the talus measured?

By observing the width of the joint space between the talus and medial malleolus.

In normality, this space between talus and medial malleolus is equal to which other space?

The space in the weight bearing part of the joint between talus and lower tibia.

Treatment of Fracture of the Lateral Malleolus with Lateral Displacement of the Talus

How are these fractures reduced?

By strong inward pressure on the lateral malleolus.

How is the fracture held reduced?

By a below-knee plaster cast with a heel support or by internal fixation.

For how long does the cast normally remain?

About eight weeks.

Should the fracture re-displace inside the cast, what treatment would you recommend?

The lateral malleolus should be screwed.

The screw passes from where to where?

From the outer part of the lateral malleolus through the lateral malleolus and well into the tibia, or for spiral fractures transfixion screws through fragments only.

After operation, for how long should a plaster be worn?

Eight weeks.

When is weight bearing permitted?

After two weeks approximately.

Fractures of Both Malleoli with Displacement of Talus

How is this produced?

By an abduction or lateral rotation force.

Since both malleoli are fractured, what treatment would you recommend?

Operation is usually advised.

Do we usually screw both malleoli in these cases?

No, usually the medial malleolus is transfixed and this automatically holds the talus and lateral malleolus correctly.

If the medial malleolus is held in the correct position with a screw, why should this guarantee that the talus and lateral malleolus will come into correct position?

Because the medial and lateral ligaments are intact.

Sometimes the lateral malleolus is also transfixed with a screw and this depends on .... preference.

The surgeon's.

How long after operation is the cast retained?

About ten weeks.

When is walking usually permitted with this type of fracture?

About three weeks after the operation.

Diastasis of Inferior Tibiofibular Joint

What sort of injury produces this diastasis?

A violent abduction injury that is withstood by the lateral malleolus.

If the lateral malleolus can tolerate this stress, the full brunt of the force therefore falls heavily on the .... joint.

Inferior tibiofibular.

With this injury, what happens to the talus?

The talus is shifted laterally.

What happens to the medial ligament?

It is either ruptured or it avulses the medial malleolus.

With this diastatis of inferior tibiofibular joint, where else might one see a fracture?

The fibula is usually fractured high up often near the knee joint.

With diastasis of the inferior tibiofibular joint, is it best to treat in a plaster conservatively or to put a screw across the diastasis?

Closed reduction is notoriously difficult and screw fixation of the inferior tibiofibular joint is recommended.

The screw passes transversely from the ..... to the ..... .

Fibula.
Tibia.

If the diastasis is complicated with the fracture of the medial malleolus, what would you do about that?

Transfix medial malleolus with a screw.

How long is the plaster retained after this operation?

For eight weeks.

When is walking permitted?

After two or three weeks.

When dealing with diastasis of inferior tibiofibular joint, occasionally the fracture may spring back spontaneously into a normal looking position. Why should an X-ray of the whole fibula be taken if there be any doubt about the diastasis of the inferior tibiofibular joint?

Because almost invariably a fracture will be located in the fibula in one part or other of its length.

Which figure in the enclosure indicates a diastasis of inferior tibiofibular joint?

Diagram 5.

Posterior Marginal Fracture of Tibia

Which diagrams indicate this type of fracture in the enclosure?

Diagrams 6 and 12.

How is this fracture sustained?

If a force pushes the tibia forward while the foot is anchored to the ground, then a triangle of the posterior part of the tibia can be sheared off as it impinges on the talus.

Usually this fracture is associated with two other fractures. What are they?

1. Fracture of medial malleolus.
2. Fracture of lateral malleolus.

Is it rare to get a posterior tibial marginal fracture on its own?

Yes.

Since both malleoli may be fractured, name two forces that can produce this injury resulting in the marginal fracture of the tibia.

1. An abduction rotation injury.
2. An adduction injury.

The small triangular fragment of tibia is displaced in which direction?

Upwards.

What does this do to the articular surface of the lower tibia?

Puts a step in it.

Is the triangular fragment of tibia usually small or large?

Usually small.

If the fragment of tibia is very large, it has to be restored ..... in order to avoid the later complication of ..... .

Perfectly.
Osteoarthritis.

Treatment of Posterior Marginal Fracture of Tibia

If the fragment is small, what do we do?

Ignore the tibial fragment if it is small and treat the medial and lateral malleolar fracture as indicated above.

How is a larger triangular tibia fracture held correctly?

With the aid of a transfixing screw.

After this operation, how long would you retain
a plaster cast?

Ten weeks.

Vertical Compression Fracture of the Tibia

What diagrams in the enclosure represent this
type of fracture?

Diagrams 13 and 14.

This injury is usually caused by a fall from a
height. What other bone in the region of the
ankle is fractured by a fall from a height?

Classically the calcaneus.

Which is the commoner, fracture of the calcaneus
or fracture of the vertical compression type of
the tibia?

Fracture of the calcaneus.

Name two types of vertical compression fracture
of the tibia.

1. Anterior marginal fracture of the tibia plus
   anterior shift of the talus.
2. Comminuted fracture of tibial articular surface plus fracture of the fibula and upward
   displacement of the talus.

Treatment of Vertical Compression Fracture of the Tibia

If the ankle is violently disorganized and there
are many tiny pieces of bone from tibia, fibula
and talus, it is best to do what operation?

Arthrodesis of the ankle joint as a primary procedure should be considered.

With a completely disorganized ankle in an
elderly person suffering from a vertical compression fracture, what treatment would you
suggest?

Plaster immobilization and simply accept the
disorganized state of affairs.

With fractures that are less severe and when only
one or two large fragments are to be replaced,
how would you proceed?

Internal fixation of large fragments is worthwhile in this situation.

CHAPTER 25

SOFT TISSUE INJURIES ABOUT THE ANKLE

Rupture of the Lateral Ligaments of the Ankle

Name the three important lateral ligaments of the ankle.

1. Anterior talofibular ligament.
2. The posterior talofibular ligament.
3. Calcaneofibular ligament.

What sort of force would rupture the lateral ligaments?

An adduction force may cause complete rupture.

What happens to the talus in complete rupture?

The talus is tilted over so that superior articulating surface comes in contact with the fibular articulating surface.

In effect, the talus is subluxated within the .... mortise.

Tibio-Fibular.

The patient gives a history of an ..... injury.

Adduction.

Severe pain, swelling and bruising are noted in the ..... aspect of the ankle.

Lateral.

* How does one distinguish between a simple strain of the lateral ligament and a complete rupture of the lateral ligaments?

X-ray the ankle with antero-postero views while an adduction force is applied to the heel.

Does this require an anaesthetic?

Yes.

If, indeed, the two ligaments are completely ruptured, the talus is shown to be ..... medially.

Tilted.

What significance do you attach to a twenty degree tilt of the talus whilst applying an adduction force to the heel under general anaesthetic?

A twenty degree tilt is not necessarily abnormal.

What would you do to see if this degree of tilt is normal for this patient?

Do a similar manipulation with the good ankle and see if it tilts twenty degrees or so as the involved ankle did.

How do you treat rupture of the lateral ligaments of the ankle?

Six weeks in a below-knee plaster cast is essential.

What surgical procedure might be carried out?

Some surgeons prefer to suture the torn capsule and ligaments to be sure the frayed ends are apposed.

Should the ankle be protected in plaster after operation?

Yes, for 6 weeks.

If one has made a misdiagnosis and has mistaken a simple strain for a complete rupture, what is the main complication in the years to come?

Recurrent subluxation of the ankle may ensue.

CHAPTER 26

RUPTURE OF THE CALCANEAL TENDON

* What is the other name for this tendon?

Tendo achilles.

Is the rupture complete or incomplete in most cases?

Always complete.

* Where does the tendon rupture?

About two inches (5 cm) above its insertion.

* What is the main symptom of calcaneal tendon rupture?

A sudden severe pain at the back of the ankle associated with a feeling that the back of the ankle has been struck: usually the patient is jumping or running at the time.

* What is the main finding on physical examination?

Extreme tenderness at the site of the rupture. A gap can be felt along the tendon about two inches above its insertion.

What happens to the motor power of the foot?

This is reduced so far as plantar flexion is concerned.

Name three muscle groups that can continue to plantar flex the foot but rather weakly.

1. Tibialis posterior.
2. Peronei.
3. Toe flexors.

Don't be deceived by the retention of some plantar flexion capacity after rupture of the ..... tendon.

Achilles.

Treatment of Calcaneal Tendon Rupture

* Give two.

1. Conservative treatment consists of plaster immobilization with knee flexed to ninety degrees and ankle in full plantar flexion for five weeks.
2. Operative repair of the severed tendon using stainless steel wire is reserved usually for young athletes.

* With operation, is plaster immobilization still necessary?

Yes, the knee must be held at right angled flexion and moderate ankle plantar flexion for four weeks.

* A common injury that might simulate an achilles tendon rupture is that of rupture of the ..... tendon.

Plantaris.

* During what activity is the plantaris ruptured?

With forceful plantar flexion as in running up steps the plantaris might rupture.

* What does the patient hear and feel during this incident?

The patient feels extreme pain in the calf and hears a crack that makes him feel he has been hit by a stone.

117

* What is the common finding on palpation of plantaris rupture?

A very tender plantaris muscle situated at about mid-calf level.

* With rupture of plantaris tendon, which movement of the ankle is extremely painful?

Dorsi flexion.

* How is ruptured plantaris treated?

Heat, crepe bandage, non-weight bearing on crutches for two weeks and rest.

CHAPTER 27

FRACTURES OF THE CALCANEUS, TALUS, TARSAL BONES, METATARSALS AND PHALANGES

* How are fractures of the calcaneus sustained?

Fall from a height.

* Which is the more common — a compression injury that crushes the subtalar joint or an isolated crack in the tuberosity?

The compression injury is more common and more serious.

Minor Fracture without Compression

* What is the usual history?

A fall of a few feet on to the heel.

* What is the main complaint?

Severe localized pain in the heel plus bruising and inability to walk.

* Physical examination reveals two outstanding features. What are they?

1. Marked local tenderness.
2. Ecchymosis on the sole of the foot.

* In the diagnosis, a special radiographic view is essential in order not to miss this fracture. What is it?

An axial view is essential with the foot fully dorsi flexed. In this way, the tuberosity fracture is easily seen.

* How would you treat the isolated crack fracture of the tuberosity?

Four weeks in a below-knee plaster cast with a heel, or crepe bandage, ice pack, and elevate limb.

Are there any complications?

Rarely.

Compression Fracture of Calcaneus

Why is this a serious injury?

Because there is always permanent impairment of foot function.

What is the main physical finding on examination?

A broadening of the heel area as seen from behind.

* Which movement is the most restricted following this fracture?

Inversion and eversion at the subtalar joint are grossly restricted.

Apart from the subtalar, which other joint is involved in this compression fracture?

The calcaneal-cuboid joint is often involved.

* What other bone might be fractured at a higher level by a fall onto the feet from a height?

Compression fracture of a vertebral body is common, e.g. T12.

On the radiograph, there is one striking feature seen in the lateral view. What is it?

The tuberosity-joint angle normally forty degrees is flattened and so reduced to 0 degrees, in many cases.

Treatment of these Calcaneal Fractures

* After this type of fracture, namely a compression fracture of the calcaneus, is the foot ever restored to normal?

No.

* The fragmentation of the subtalar joint almost certainly gives rise ultimately to ..... Osteoarthritis.

* The standard method of treatment of these fractures then is to accept the subtalar disruption and go for active exercises. In the early painful stage, the foot might be elevated on a ..... frame.

Braun's.

What is the point in elevating the foot?

To eliminate foot oedema.

During this passive stage of rest, exercises should be undertaken to which joints? Give three.

1. The ankle joint.
2. The subtalar joint.
3. The midtarsal joint.

In which of these joints would you expect there to be extreme discomfort and restriction of movement? Give two.

1. The subtalar joint.
2. The midtarsal joint.

* For how long would you confine the patient to bed?

Three or four weeks.

If the patient gets up and about too early, what might happen to the foot?

Gravitational oedema may be a hindrance to restoration of movement.

If you had a patient with severe pain that went on for three months after the fracture, what treatment surgically may you recommend?

Arthrodesis of the subtalar joint, or triple arthrodesis.

What is meant by closed reduction?

An attempt is made to compress the lateral spread and using a posterior spike, reduce the upward displacement of the back of the heel.

Complications

Name two joints that are stiffened by this fracture.

1. The subtalar joint.
2. The midtarsal joint.

How may this joint stiffening be minimised?

By elevating the foot and doing active exercises early on.

Name another complication of this fracture.

Osteoarthritis of the subtalar joint.

How is this condition best treated when it is associated with severe pain and restriction of the subtalar joint?

Arthrodesis of the subtalar joint and perhaps of the midtarsal joint.

Another complication is a limp. What is the mechanics of this?

The fracture is such that the achilles tendon insertion is shifted proximally as the calcaneus is flattened and so the calf muscles are made unduly slack giving rise to a loss of spring in the gait, during step-off.

As mentioned above, there is another bone that might be fractured at the same time as the calcaneus. What is it?

A vertebral body crush fracture in the lower thoracic spine is quite common.

How would you diagnose it?

By clinical examination and radiologically.

Fractures of the Talus

* Whereabouts in the talus are most serious fractures located?

In the neck of the bone.

* What are the other types of fractures seen in the talus?

1. Fracture of body of talus.
2. Chipped or flaked fractures from an articular surface.

Fracture of the Neck of the Talus

What is the commonest mechanism of this injury?

A violent force directed upwards against the middle of the sole of the foot fractures the narrow neck of the talus just in front of the body of the bone.

In what direction is the body of the talus dislocated?

Backwards out of the ankle mortise and downwards.

Treatment of Fracture of the Neck of the Talus

Why is reduction urgent?

Because the skin stretched over talus soon necroses.

How is the fracture reduced? Give two methods.

1. By manipulation.
2. By operation and internal fixation with Kirschner wires.

How is it held in position?

By a below-knee plaster until fracture is united (eight weeks).

How does one achieve maximum stability of the fracture?

Occasionally by holding the foot in equinus, i.e. plantar flexion.

How long would you leave the foot in equinus?

For three weeks.

What might happen if you leave it longer than three weeks?

The foot may stay in equinus permanently.

When the three weeks in equinus is up, what then?

Immobilise for further five weeks in neutral position.

Complications of Fracture of Neck of Talus

Give two.

1. Non-union.
2. Avascular necrosis.

Non-union is frequently associated with what condition?

Avascular necrosis of the proximal body fragment.

Why does the body of talus undergo necrosis?

Due to damage to the nutrient vessels.

Which carpal bone fracture is similar to the talus by virtue of this unusual blood supply?

Fracture of scaphoid in wrist.

How would you diagnose avascular necrosis of the talus?

By the eighth week after the injury, the difference in radiographic density is noted. The bone scan clinches it.

Does the dead bone appear more dense or less dense than the rest of the bones of the foot?

More dense.

121

Treatment of Avascular Necrosis and Non-union

The aim of the operation is to eliminate which three joints?

1. The ankle joint.
2. The subtalar joint.
3. Talonavicular joint by arthrodesis.

What would you do if avascular necrosis has led to collapse and disintegration of the body of the talus?

It would then be necessary to fuse the tibia to the calcaneus after excising the dead talus.

How would you treat osteoarthritis following fracture of the neck of the talus?

Osteoarthritis of the ankle and the subtalar joints is almost inevitable after avascular necrosis of the body of the talus, so the only procedure that could be done is to carry out an arthrodesis from tibia to the calcaneus after excising the dead talus.

How would you fill in this gap?

By a square or rectangle of iliac crest bone.

Fractures of the Metatarsal Bones and Phalanges of the Toes

How are most metatarsal fractures produced?

By direct violence from a heavy object falling upon the foot.

Is fracture of the 5th metatarsal base common or rare?

Common.

How is it produced?

By twisting injury in which the foot is forced into inversion and equinus.

In an avulsion fracture, the base of the metatarsal bone is pulled off by which tendon?

Peroneus brevis tendon.

What is the main physical sign in a fracture of the 5th metatarsal bone?

Tenderness at the base of the 5th metatarsal.

Why is a below-knee walking plaster preferred to strapping?

Because it relieves the pain more effectively.

For how long would you retain the cast?

Three weeks.

What treatment would you recommend after removal of the cast?

Physiotherapy, active exercises and heat.

Fractures of Metatarsal Shafts

How is this sustained?

By a heavy object falling on the foot.

What types of fractures are there? Give two.

1. Transverse.
2. Short oblique.

Do these fractures heal readily?

Yes.

Treatment of Fractures of Metatarsal Shafts

Why is this fracture immobilized?

Mainly for the relief of pain — union will occur in any event.

For how long would you recommend the plaster be applied?

Three weeks.

What is the extent of the plaster?

From below-knee to metatarsal head with ankle at a right angle.

Fractures of the Phalanges of the Toes

How are phalangeal fractures sustained?

Usually by a crushing injury.

Which toe is the commonest?

The great toe.

How do you treat a fracture of a phalanx?

After the swelling has subsided, the fractured toe can be strapped to the adjacent toe and protected with a wooden splint to prevent impact against other objects.

CHAPTER 28

OSTEOARTHRITIS

General Considerations

* Osteoarthritis is a joint condition character-ised by increasing pain, stiffness and deform-ity.

* Give three other names for osteoarthritis.

1. Hypertrophic arthritis.
2. Degenerative arthritis.
3. Osteoarthrosis.

* O.A. is equal to ....

Old age.

* O.A. is equal to ..... .

Osteoarthritis.

* Osteoarthritis is usually caused by ..... and ..... .

Wear.
Tear.

* If a joint was never put under ....., it would never become osteoarthritic.

Stress.

* What is the commonest predisposing factor to osteoarthritis?

Old age.

* Think of another one starting with "O".

Obesity.

Give two ways in which injury can predispose to osteoarthritis.

1. A fracture into the joint can roughen the usually smooth surfaces.
2. A torn cartilage can do likewise.

Name four diseases that predispose to osteo-arthritis.

1. Perthes' disease.
2. Slipped upper femoral epiphysis.
3. Rheumatoid arthritis.
4. Haemophilia.

* Name a type of malalignment of a joint that may predispose to osteoarthritis.

Bow leg.

* In summary, give six predisposing causes of osteoarthritis.

1. Old age.
2. Obesity.
3. Fracture into the joint.
4. Torn cartilage or loose body.
5. Previous disease/rheumatoid arthritis or haemophilia or septic arthritis.
6. Malalignment.

What is meant by primary osteoarthritis?

It is primary when there is no obvious cause.

Pathology

* Give three pathological changes seen in an osteoarthritic joint.

1. The articular cartilage (not the meniscus) is slowly worn away.
2. Bare bone is seen underneath it (eburnation).
3. The bony build-up on the sides of the joint adjacent to this is known as osteophyte formation.

Clinical Features

* Most patients with osteoarthritis are old/young.

Old.

* When osteoarthritis occurs in young patients, it is usually secondary to ..... or ..... .

Injury; Disease.
e.g.: Injury — fracture into joint.
         Disease — Perthes' disease of the hip joint.

* The symptoms are P.A.L.S.

Pain
Altered position (deformity at a later stage).
Limp in lower limb (osteoarthritis).
Stiffness.

* On examination of any joint, we make four observations. What are they?

1. Inspection.
2. Palpation.
3. Move.
4. X-ray.

* Looking at the arthritic joint, we may see ..... .

Deformity.

On feeling the joint, we might feel ....

Bony thickening (there is usually no increased warmth on feeling).

* On testing for movement, we see ..... or ..... restriction.

Slight; Marked.
(according to degree of arthritis).

* In addition to inspection, palpation, move, X-ray, we might add ..... .

Hearing. In severe arthritis, a grinding crepitation might be heard.

* X-ray findings. On the X-ray, the joint space is narrowed. Why?

Because the articular cartilage has worn away.

* The bone under the articular cartilage becomes ..... .

Sclerotic, i.e. dense.

* At the edge of the joint, the bone proliferates and this can be seen on the X-ray as ....

Osteophyte formation.

Radiographic Examination

* Name three features seen on the radiographs of an osteoarthritic joint.

1. The diminution of cartilage space.
2. Sclerosis of bone under the cartilage.
3. Lipping of the joint margins due to osteophyte formation.

Differential Diagnosis

* Usually there are three main features that distinguish osteoarthritis from inflammatory forms of arthritis. What are they?

With osteoarthritis there is:
1. No synovial thickening.
2. No increased local warmth.
3. No muscle spasm.

* What happens to the E.S.R. with osteoarthritis?

It is not increased as with other forms of arthritis.

* The main radiographic difference between inflammatory arthritis and osteoarthritis is what?

On the radiographs there is sclerosis with osteoarthritis and rarefaction with inflammatory arthritic disease.

Treatment of Osteoarthritis

* The treatment of osteoarthritis may be classified into two groups. What are they?

1. Conservative treatment.
2. Operative treatment.

* Name two types of physiotherapy that might help.

1. Local heat.
2. Muscle strengthening exercises.

* Name two anti-inflammatory drugs that might help relieve the pain of osteoarthritis.

1. Butazolidine — (Phenylbutazone).
2. Indocid — (Indomethacin).

* Give two other conservative methods of treating osteoarthritis.

1. Hydrocortisone injection into the joint.
2. Supportive bandage or appliance.

* When the disability is severe, there are two possible types of operation that might be used to help. What are they?

1. Arthroplasty.
2. Arthrodesis.

* What is meant by arthroplasty?

This is the re-fashioning of a joint.

* What is meant by arthrodesis?

This is the elimination of a joint by fusion of the bone ends.

* Name two types of arthroplasty.

1. Reconstructive arthroplasty, e.g. Charnley's total hip replacement.
2. Excision arthroplasty such as Girdlestone's operation.

CHAPTER 29

ANKYLOSING SPONDYLITIS

Definition of ankylosing spondylitis.

This is a chronic inflammatory condition of the spine and sacro-iliac joints associated with pain and stiffness in the back with occasional peripheral joint involvement.

* These two words mean inflammation of the spine progressing to ..... obliteration.

Joint.

Is there a genetic predisposition to ankylosing spondylitis?

Yes — it is much commoner in family members than in the general population.

* Is the condition commoner in men or women?

Men.

* Is it commoner in the older age group or in the young?

Young people between 15 and 25 are more commonly affected.

* In which joints does it usually commence?

Sacro-iliac joint or thoraco-lumbar joints.

What is HLA—B27?

An antigen found in 90 per cent of sufferers of ankylosing spondylitis.

Is HLA—B27 present in all patients with ankylosing spondylitis?

No, it is present in 90 per cent of patients.

Name the three pathological changes which are seen in order of development in ankylosing spondylitis.

1. Infiltration of round cells with granulation tissue formation and erosion of adjacent bone takes place in the joints.
2. Replacement of granulation tissue with fibrous tissue.
3. Ossification of the fibrous tissue.

Do all people with the antigen HLA—B27 in their blood stream develop ankylosing spondylitis?

No, only a small percentage do so.

* In the early stages, there is inflammation of the tissues of the joint and then finally the condition goes on to cause complete joint ..... with the growth of ..... right through the joint.

Obliteration; Bone.

* In the early stages, the joints appear to be ..... and later the whole spine radiologically is seen to be ossified and the condition radiologically is then called a ..... spine.

Calcified.

Bamboo.

* If the costo-vertebral joints are involved, the patient has difficulty with ..... .

Breathing.

* In cases of bamboo spine, there is usually a marked ..... in the thoracic spine.

Kyphosis.

* What are the early symptoms of which the patient complains?

A jarring pain in the low back, going on to a feeling of stiffness in the whole spine.

* Ankylosing spondylitis then is a chronic inflammation progressing slowly into bony ankylosis of the joints of the spinal column and occasionally involving the major ..... joints.

Limb.

What is the prevalence of ankylosing spondylitis in Western Europe?

One in 1,000 (0.1 per cent).

* What is the cause of ankylosing spondylitis?

Unknown.

* Pathologically, there are three parts of the joint that are involved. What are they?

1. The articular cartilage.
2. The synovium.
3. The ligaments of the joint.

* On physical examination of the spine, it would be noted that all spinal movements are ..... .

Restricted.

In established cases the posture is typical — give three features.

1. Flattening of the lumbar lordosis.
2. A forward thrust of the neck.
3. Slight flexion of the hips and the knees.

* The involvement of the costo-vertebral joints gives rise to restriction of ..... expansion and this should be measured from time-to-time to observe the progress of the disease.

Chest.

Which spinal movement is the first to be affected?

A lack of extension is the earliest and the most severe disability noticed.

What is meant by Apley's wall test?

The patient is asked to stand with back to the wall: heels, buttocks, scapulae and occiput should be able to touch the wall simultaneously. If extension is seriously diminished, the patient will find this impossible.

* The early radiographs of the sacro-iliac joint show ..... and later films show these joints to be totally ..... .

Fuzziness.
Obliterated.

What is the earliest vertebral change seen on the radiographs in ankylosing spondylitis?

Flattening of the normal anterior concavity of the vertebral body.

What is the name given to this flattening of the normal anterior concavity of the vertebral body?

Squaring of the vertebral body.

* What two blood tests are significant in the diagnosis of ankylosing spondylitis?

Elevation of E.S.R. and presence of the antigen HLA—B27.

* Give four points regarding the diagnosis of ankylosing spondylitis from a clinical examination point of view and including special tests.

1. Limitation of spinal movements.
2. Reduced chest expansion.
3. Typical radiographic features of joint obliteration.
4. Raised E.S.R. and presence of HLA—B27 in the patient's blood stream.

Name six conditions that may simulate ankylosing spondylitis.

1. Reiter's disease.
2. Psoriatic arthritis.
3. Ulcerative colitis.
4. Crohn's disease.
5. Forestier's disease.
6. Behcet's syndrome.

In Reiter's disease what other two features are found?

1. Genito-urinary inflammation.
2. Ocular inflammation.

In cases of psoriatic arthritis what skin changes would you expect?

A rash and nail changes are a feature.

In ulcerative colitis ..... are found in the bowel.

Ulcerations.

Crohn's disease is also associated with bowel ..... .

Ulcers.

Give two features that are associated with Behcet's syndrome.

Buccal and genital ulcerations.

Do all these conditions share the presence of antigen HLA—B27 in the blood stream?

Yes.

What is the other name for Forestier's disease?

Ankylosing hyperostosis.

What are the two main features of Forestier's disease?

1. Common in elderly men.
2. Manifests a widespread ossification of ligament and tendon insertions.

Is the E.S.R. elevated in Forestier's disease?

No, it is normal.

Treatment of Ankylosing Spondylitis

* There was a form of treatment that had severe complications and was therefore abandoned. What was it?

Radiotherapy, in many cases, causes leukemia and radiation colitis.

* What value did radiotherapy have?

It gave relief from pain and occasionally arrested the disease.

* Modern treatment consists of three measures, what are they?

1. Vigorous spinal exercises together with deep breathing exercises to prevent forward flexion and stiffness of costo-vertebral joints.
2. Anti-inflammatory drugs such as
   (a) Indomethacin and
   (b) Phenylbutazone.
3. Sleeping on the back on a hard bed is thought to prevent flexion deformity.

* What can be done surgically for the established condition of ankylosing spondylitis?

Spinal wedge osteotomy can be carried out on lumbar or cervical regions in severe cases when the flexion deformity is crippling.

What does this achieve?

In the cervical region the wedge resection enables the patient to look directly ahead instead of looking at the floor — likewise with the lumbar spine, the patient is straightened up.

How may ankylosing spondylitis of the hips be treated?

By total hip replacement.

CHAPTER 30

GOUTY ARTHRITIS AND BURSITIS

Define gout.

Gout manifests as recurrent attacks of acute synovitis associated with disordered purine metabolism.

* Gout is a clinical manifestation of a disturbed ..... metabolism.

Purine.

* Gout is characterised by deposition of .... salts such as .... in the joints or in the ear, the walls of bursae and ligaments.

Uric acid; Sodium biurate.

* Cause of gout?

Unknown.

* Does heredity play a part? Yes or No.

Yes.

* Name two drinks that might predispose to an attack of gout in susceptible people.

Heavy wines and beer.

* Name three purine-rich foods that may bring on an attack of gout in a susceptible person.

1. Liver.
2. Sweetbread (pancreas).
3. Meat — beef or lamb.

* May injury to a joint precipitate an attack? Yes or No.

Yes.

* In gout, which acid may be increased in the blood stream?

Uric acid.

* Why does this acid increase in the blood?

Because of impaired excretion of uric acid by the kidneys or by increased uric acid production.

* What is the normal blood uric acid in the Solin method?

2.0 — 7.0 mgs per 100 mls.

* What is the name of the salt deposited in connective tissues in the case of gout?

Sodium biurate.

* Why are the salts deposited commonly in the articular cartilage of the joints of the foot?

Because the blood supply is sluggish in that area.

* What is primary gout and how prevalent is it?

An inherited disorder with over-production or under-excretion of uric acid. 95% of cases are primary.

Give an example of secondary gout.

Renal failure causing under-excretion of uric acid.

* The deposits set up an inflammatory reaction which is possibly ..... in nature.

Autoimmune.

* In acute gout, the deposit of sodium biurate is ..... and is soon reabsorbed.

Microscopic.

* The rapid reabsorption returns the joint to ..... .

Normal.

* In chronic gout, name three parts of the joint involved.

1. The menisci of the knee.
2. Ligaments of the joints.
3. Articular ends of bones.

* The joint becomes permanently ..... in chronic gout.

Disorganised.

* Name two other sites where gouty deposits might be seen, apart from the joints.

1. Olecranon bursa.
2. In the cartilage of the ear.

* What is the name of the nodular deposits of sodium biurate?

Tophi.

Clinical Features of Gout

* Is it more common in women than men?

No, much more common in men.

* Is it commoner over forty or under forty?

Usually over forty years of age.

* Which is the commonest joint in the body to be involved?

The great toe joint (metatarso-phalangeal).

* When we examine a joint, we make four observations. What are they?

1. Inspection.
2. Palpation.
3. Move.
4. X-ray.

* When we inspect, what do we see with gout in the toe?

A swollen, red, shiny joint.

* Palpation?

Excruciating tenderness and warmth.

* Movements?

Restricted and painful.

* X-ray?

Nil in early stages. Subchondral cyst formation is seen on the X-ray in the later stages.

* The cysts seen in the later stage on X-ray are due to?

Sodium biurate deposits.

* Which bursa is commonly affected with gout?

Olecranon bursa.

* What are the lumps that might be felt in the olecranon bursa called?

Tophi.

* To investigate gout, what two blood tests would you do?

1. Serum uric acid content.
2. White cell count (usually raised).

* Name three conditions that can simulate gout in that they produce a sudden onset of acute joint pain?

1. Pyogenic arthritis.
2. Haemophilic arthritis.
3. Rheumatic fever.

* What features suggest gout? Name four.

1. History of previous attacks.
2. Raised blood uric acid content.
3. Tophi in the ears or elsewhere.
4. Recovery with the use of Colchicine.

Course of the Disease

* In acute gout, the joint returns quickly to ..... .

Normal.

131

* In chronic gout, however, permanent joint disorganisation is ..... .

Inevitable.

Treatment of Gout

* Name four drugs used in the treatment of gout.

1. Zyloprim (Allopurinol).
2. Colchicine.
3. Butazolidine-Phenylbutazone.
4. Indomethacin.

* Colchicine is given every three hours until the pain ..... .

Disappears.

* A complication of Colchicine is ..... .

Diarrhoea.

Give the doses of the two drugs most effective in acute gout.

1. Indomethacin 50 mg, six hourly.
2. Phenylbutazone 200 mg, six hourly.

* What are the other names for gouty arthritis? Give two.

1. Podagra.
2. Urate crystal synovitis.

* What metabolic disorder gives rise to gout?

It is due to disturbed purine metabolism.

* What is the name of the salt that is deposited in various parts of the body in this condition?

Sodium biurate.

* Give four possible sites where the uric acid salts (biurates) are deposited.

1. Cartilage of joints.
2. Cartilage of ear.
3. Walls of bursae.
4. Ligaments.

Cause of Gouty Arthritis

* The precise cause of the disturbance of metabolism is .... .

Unknown.

* Is there an inherited predisposition?

Yes.

* In susceptible persons, there are several factors that might induce an attack. Give four such factors.

Excessive consumption of:
1. Beer.
2. Heavy wines.
3. A recent injury.
4. An operation.

Pathology of Gouty Arthritis

* What is the primary fault?

Impaired excretion of uric acid by the kidneys or increased urate production.

* What happens to the urate level in the serum?

It may be increased.

* What is the normal serum uric acid in milligrams?

2.0 to 7.0 milligrams per 100 mls.

* In the blood, the uric acid is in solution in a loose combination with ..... .

Proteins.

* When uric acid comes out of solution, it forms a salt called ....

Sodium biurate.

* The sodium biurate is deposited in the form of ..... in certain connective tissues.

Crystals.

* Why do the crystals composed of sodium biurate deposit in articular cartilage or synovial tissue?

Because these tissues are easily injured and because they have a sluggish blood supply.

* What effect do the deposited crystals have on the tissues.

They cause inflammation.

* With acute gout, how large is the deposit of sodium biurate?

It is microscopic.

* With chronic gout, however, there are widespread deposits of ....

Sodium biurate. These occur in the joint cartilages, ligaments and articular ends of bones.

* What is the other name for a gouty deposit?

Tophus.

* Name two other sites where tophi might occur.

1. Olecranon bursa.
2. In the cartilage of the ear.

Clinical Features of Gouty Arthritis

* Is the condition common in men or women?

Men.

* Is it common in the over forties or under forties?

Over forties.

* Name the peripheral joints that are involved in gouty arthritis. Give four.

1. Toe joints.
2. Tarsal joints.
3. Ankle joints.
4. Small joints of the hand.

* Where is the first attack usually?

In the region of the great toe.

* Give four clinical features of the toe joint which is involved in gouty arthritis.

1. The joint is very red.
2. It is swollen.
3. The skin is shiny.
4. It is extremely painful.

* What happens to the movements in gouty arthritis?

Movements are very restricted.

* How long does an acute attack usually last?

One to four days.

* Is the joint normal between attacks?

Yes.

* In chronic gout, how many joints might be involved?

Many.

Bursitis – Gouty Bursitis

* Which is the most commonly affected bursa?

Olecranon bursa.

* On palpating the olecranon bursa, two features might be noted. What are they?

Fluid and uric acid aggregations may be present.

* What is the other name for uric acid aggregations?

Tophi.

* Where else might uric acid salts be seen?

In the ear cartilages.

* In acute gout, what radiographic changes are seen?

None.

* In chronic gout, how do deposits of uric acid salts manifest radiologically?

As clearcut erosions adjacent to the joint.

* Name three blood picture changes that might be detected in acute gouty arthritis.

1. Plasma — uric acid elevated.
2. E.S.R. — elevated.
3. White cell count — elevated.

* What might aspiration of an involved joint yield?

A small quantity of turbid fluid but never organisms.

* What would microscopic examination of the synovial fluid reveal?

Biurate crystals.

* Give three conditions that may simulate acute gout.

1. Acute septic arthritis.
2. Haemophilic arthritis.
3. Rheumatic fever.

* Give six features that would distinguish gout from the abovementioned conditions.

In gout we see:
1. History of previous attacks.
2. Symptom-free interval.
3. Raised serum urate content.
4. Tophi in ears or elsewhere.
5. Crystals in synovial fluid.
6. Favourable response to treatment.

* Chronic gout involving several joints may simulate ....

Rheumatoid arthritis.

Treatment of Gout

* How do you treat the joint itself with acute gout?

By resting it in a splint.

* In chronic gout, several drugs may be used to reduce plasma urate level. Name two drugs used in this connection.

1. Probenecid.
2. Allopurinol (Zyloprim).

* How does Probenecid act?

It reduces renal tubular reabsorption of urates and thus increases their excretion in the urine.

* How does Allopurinol work?

It reduces the formation of uric acid by inhibiting the enzyme xanthine oxidase.

* Why is Allopurinol safer than Probenecid?

Allopurinol is safer because it does not increase the load of urate in the kidneys with the associated hazard of stone formation.

Apart from urate salts being deposited in the tissues and joints, what other salts mght be found there?

Calcium pyrophosphate.

Calcification then of menisci or articular cartilage is seen radiologically due to these calcium pyrophosphate salts and this condition is known as ....

Pseudo gout.

How would you treat pseudo gout? Give three methods.

1. By resting the joint.
2. Aspiration of joint fluid.
3. Give Phenylbutazone tablets (butazolidine) or Indocid.

Pseudo gout is characterized then by crystals of .... deposited in the cartilage of menisci of ..... .

Calcium pyrophosphate.
Joints.

CHAPTER 31

PAGET'S DISEASE

* Define Paget's disease.

A painful disease of obscure origin affecting one or more bones with a gradual progression resulting in a thickened, spongy and deformed condition of the involved bone or bones.

* What is another name for Paget's disease?

Osteitis Deformans.

* Does it involve usually one bone or more than one bone?

Usually more than one bone.

* What are the three main features of the Paget bone?

1. The bone is hot.
2. Thick.
3. Bent.

* Why is it hot?

Because of increased blood supply.

* Why is it thick?

Because of hypertrophy of the cortical layer.

* Why is it bent, in the case of long bones?

Because, during the soft phase, the bone bends and stays bent after it has hardened up.

* So when we see a tibia, for example, that looks bent and feels to be thick and hot, we think of ..... disease.

Paget's.

* Name one other disease that was described by Sir James Paget.

Paget's disease of the breast (a type of carcinoma).

* What is the cause of Paget's disease?

Unknown, perhaps a viral infection.

* Is Paget's disease of bone rare or common?

Common.

Name three countries where it is common.

In Australia, Britain and Germany, more than 3% of people over 40 have Paget's disease.

* Name the most commonly affected bones.

Pelvis, femur, tibia, skull and vertebrae.

* Is the disease sometimes confined to one bone?

Yes.

* Usually, however, it spreads to involve ..... bones.

Other.

* During the "soft" stage, the cortex of the bone loses its compact density and becomes ..... .

Spongy.

* Since bone is laid down on the inside and the outside of the cortex, the bone as a whole becomes ..... .

Thicker.

* Usually there is a sharp distinction between cortex and medulla in the normal bone, but with Paget's disease, this sharp distinction is ..... .

Lost.

* The spaces become filled with ..... tissue.

Fibrous.

* In the later stages, the bones tend to become very hard and from a surgeon's point of view, this poses a particular problem. What is it?

When pinning a fracture, the bone might be too hard to get a drill or pin into it.

* Name three complications of Paget's disease of bone.

1. Pathological fracture.
2. High output cardiac failure.
3. Osteosarcoma.

Skull enlargement may result in four changes.

1. Bigger hat required.
2. Headaches.
3. Deafness.
4. Blindness.

Clinical Features of Paget's Disease

* Does it occur before or after the age of forty in most cases?

After the age of forty.

* Sometimes a routine radiographic examination will pick up asymptomatic ..... disease.

Paget's.

* Name two symptoms you might expect from the patient with a femur that manifests a hot, thick, bent bone.

1. Pain in the bone.
2. Shortening due to the bowing.

* When Paget's disease involves the skull, the patient may have to get a larger size of ..... .

Hat.

What does Paget's disease do to the spine?

It produces kyphosis and thus shortening of the patient plus spinal stenosis and low back pain.

* As the skull bones enlarge, the foramina may get smaller and thus occlude certain nerves such as the 8th nerve, giving rise to ..... .

Deafness.

* When the femur or tibia bends, in which direction does the bone bow?

Anteriorly and laterally.

From the pathology mentioned above, you can deduce what the radiographic findings would be. Name five.

1. Thickening of the bone mainly from widening of the cortex — the cortex is widened by increase in bone on its inner and on its outer sides.
2. The cortex assumes a cotton-wool appearance, due to loss of density.
3. There is marked coarsening of the bone trabeculae.
4. In the later stages, there is increased density of the affected bone.
5. The long bones are bent as well as thickened.

What urine changes are observed?

Urine hydroxyproline is increased.

Blood Tests

* Name two blood tests that you would expect to be abnormal.

The alkaline phosphatase content of the serum is increased as is the plasma hydroxyproline.

* Are these the only constant serological changes seen in Paget's disease?

Yes.

Treatment

* Name three drugs that might be of value in the treatment of Paget's disease.

1. Fluoride compounds.
2. Calcitonin.
3. Diphosphonates.

* Are there any indications for surgery? Give two.

1. Fractures in a Pagety bone require internal fixation.
2. Severe bowing in a Pagety bone may require osteotomy to straighten it followed by internal fixation with a plate or Huckstep nail.

* Finally, on Paget's disease of bone, when the disease is widespread the increased blood supply to the involved bone is such that the patient may manifest the symptoms of an .... fistula.

Arterio-venous.

* This arterio-venous fistula, of course, can have a very detrimental effect on ..... function.

Heart.

* How?

It may produce high output cardiac failure.

CHAPTER 32

RICKETS – COELIAC, NUTRITIONAL, RENAL AND VITAMIN RESISTANT

What is the other name for Coeliac Rickets?

Gluten-induced Rickets.

The Coeliac disease is a digestive disorder, characterized by malabsorption of ..... .

Fat.

As a result of this malabsorption, there is excess fat in the ..... .

Stools.

Before knowledge was gained as to control of the disease, it was often complicated by ..... changes in the bones.

Rachitic.

These changes are now very rarely seen because the Coeliac disease is controllable.

Since there is malabsorption of fats, there is malabsorption of Vitamin D because Vitamin D is fat ..... .

Soluble.

The primary fault lies in the susceptibility of the ..... of the small intestine to atrophy under the influence of ..... .

Villi.
Gluten.

What is gluten?

Gluten is the protein fraction of flour.

Clinical Features of Coeliac Rickets

When does the disease of Coeliac Rickets become apparent?

In infancy or early childhood.

Since there is loss of fat in the stool and loss also of fat soluble substances in the stool, one could guess that the symptoms and signs would include such things as ..... .

Wasting.

Give five other features of Coeliac Rickets.

1. Impaired growth.
2. Failure to gain weight.
3. Muscular hypotonia.
4. Offensive stools containing twice the normal amount of fat.
5. A distended abdomen.

The skeletal changes which do not develop for several years are like those of ..... Rickets.

Infantile.

Since it is similar to Infantile Rickets, Coeliac Rickets would show a certain change in the density of the skeleton. What is it?

There is loss of density of the skeleton.

Name two changes seen in the epiphyses in Infantile Rickets.

1. The epiphyseal line is increased in depth.
2. The epiphyses are widened laterally.

The biochemical changes in the blood differ from those of Infantile Rickets. For example, the serum calcium in Coeliac Rickets is ..... . The serum phosphate is ..... or ..... .

Low.
Normal; Low.

How would one make a diagnosis of Coeliac Rickets bearing in mind that there is a malfunction of the villi of the small intestine?

By performing jejunal biopsy. This can be done with a swallowed capsule that has a special cutting device.

Treatment of Coeliac or Gluten Induced Rickets

Since the presence of gluten produces atrophy of the villi of the small intestine, treatment is to give the patient a ..... free diet.

Gluten.

In addition, there should be an abundant supply of two other substances. What are they?

1. Calcium.
2. Vitamin D.

Nutritional Rickets

In rickets, there is defective calcification of growing bone in consequence of a disturbed ..... and ..... metabolism.

Calcium.
Phosphorus.

What vitamin is deficient in nutritional rickets?

Vitamin D.

The manufacture of Vitamin D in the body is promoted by exposure to ..... .

Sunlight.

How does Vitamin D affect the calcium/phosphorus metabolism?

Vitamin D promotes the absorption of calcium and phosphorus from the intestine.

Therefore, deficiency of Vitamin D leads to inadequate absorption of ..... and ..... from the intestine.

Calcium; Phosphorus.

The level of calcium in the blood stream is maintained at the expense of the calcium in the ..... .

Skeleton.

With this lack of calcium, the osteoid in the growing epiphyses remains ..... .

Uncalcified.

Furthermore, there is a general softening of the ..... already formed.

Bones.

Clinical Features of the Nutritional Rickets

At what age does one see this disease commonly?

One year of age.

Give five signs one might see on physical examination of a child with nutritional rickets.

1. The head is large.
2. There is retarded skeletal growth.
3. The epiphyses are enlarged.
4. There is curvature of long bones.
5. There is deformity of the chest.

What does one see on the radiographs, generally speaking?

There is a general loss of density of the skeleton.

The vertical depth of the epiphyseal lines is ..... .

Increased.

Something else happens to the epiphyses. What is that?

They are widened.

Another striking feature on the radiographs is that the ends of the shafts are hollowed out and this is called ..... .

Cupping (i.e. looks like a cup).

The bones generally may undergo ..... .

Bending.

Investigations of nutritional rickets show that the serum phosphate level is usually ..... whereas the serum calcium is usually ..... .

Decreased.
Normal.

What happens, do you think, to the alkaline phosphatase in nutritional rickets?

It is increased.

The level of the alkaline phosphatase can be used as an indication of the ..... of the disease and the ..... to treatment.

Severity.
Response.

The radiographic features of nutritional rickets are so definite that a diagnosis can be made by taking an X-ray of the wrist of the patient and this will show the main features, namely?

1. Cupping of the end of the bone.
2. Increase in the depth of the epiphyseal carti-lage.
3. A reduction in the general density of the bone.

Since there are several types of rickets, the bio-chemical examination is necessary so one can assess the ....

Type of rickets.

The treatment of nutritional rickets is simply to give ....

Vitamin D.

Sometimes severe bony deformity has to be corrected by means of ..... .

Osteotomy.

There are other factors that can produce abnor-malities in the calcium phosphate metabolism. As a result, there are four other types of rickets depending on the mechanism of the calcium phosphate malfunction. Name four other types of rickets.

1. Vitamin Resistant Rickets.
2. Fanconi Syndrome.
3. Renal or Glomerular Rickets.
4. Coeliac Rickets.

Renal Rickets

What is the other name for Renal Rickets?

Glomerular rickets.

At what age do the skeletal changes become apparent?

Between five and ten years.

Why is Renal Rickets referred to as Renal Rickets?

Because the general skeletal changes are associ-ated with chronic renal impairment.

Name three pathological conditions that could cause Renal Rickets.

1. Congenital cystic changes.
2. Hydronephrosis due to ureteric obstruction.
3. Chronic nephritis.

Are the mechanics of renal deficiency leading to rachitic changes known definitely?

No.

One explanation is that malfunction of the kidneys leads to impaired excretion of ..... and as a result, there is retention of ..... in the blood.

Phosphorus.
Phosphorus.

As a result of this process, there is excess excretion of that same substance, phosphorus, in the ..... .

Intestine.

In the intestine, the phosphorus forms an insoluble compound with ..... and as a result, the calcium is not absorbed in proper ..... .

Calcium.
Amounts.

The skeletal changes consist of abnormal ..... growth and multiple bone deformities due to bone ..... .

Epiphyseal.

Softening.

In an endeavour to elevate the serum calcium, the ..... glands hypertrophy.

Parathyroid.

Clinical Features of Renal Rickets

Give two features of Renal Rickets in the child.

1. The child is of short stature.
2. The child is deformed.

The symptoms of renal failure include excessive ..... and a ..... complexion.

Thirst; Sallow.

Name three common skeletal deformities with reference to the hip, the knee and the foot regions.

1. Coxa Vara.
2. Genu Valgum (knock knees).
3. Valgus deformity of the feet.

Radiographs of sufferers of Renal Rickets show changes similar to those of Infantile Rickets (Nutritional Rickets). What are these changes?

1. Loss of density of the skeleton.
2. Depth of epiphyseal lines increased.
3. The epiphyses are widened laterally and there is cupping of the end of the shaft of the bones.
4. Bending of the bones is obvious.

Investigations of Renal Rickets

These can be calculated from the pathology.
1. The serum calcium is markedly ..... .

Depressed.

2. The serum calcium is low for reasons given above.

3. The blood urea is ..... due to kidney impairment as one would expect in chronic nephritis.

Raised.

4. Albumin is present in the ..... .

Urine.

Treatment of Renal or Glomerular Rickets consists of treating the underlying condition and in addition, the diet should be supplemented with two substances, namely ..... and ....

Calcium; Vitamin D.

Vitamin Resistant Rickets

As the name implies, this is a type of rickets that does not respond to treatment by ....

Vitamin D.

Just as in sugar diabetes, there is excess loss of sugar in the urine so with vitamin resistant rickets, there is excess loss of ..... in the urine.

Phosphate.

As a result, vitamin resistant rickets is sometimes known as ....

Chronic phosphate diabetes.

Is vitamin resistant rickets hereditary?

Yes, probably associated with a sex linked dominant gene.

The nature of the primary defect is uncertain, possibly it is a failure of reabsorption of ..... by the renal tubules or it may be a fault in the absorption of ..... from the intestines.

Phosphate.

Calcium.

At what age do the bone changes take place?

After the first year.

The biochemical changes noted include a low serum ..... level and a normal serum ..... .

Phosphate; Calcium.

The outstanding feature of vitamin resistant rickets is, of course, that the low serum phosphate level is not corrected by administration of ....

Vitamin D.

Other changes noted in the serum include elevation of the alkaline ..... .

Phosphatase.

Just as in diabetes, there is excess sugar in the urine, so with this condition of vitamin resistant rickets the urine manifests an increase or excess of ..... .

Phosphate.

It is of interest that relatives who are clinically unaffected may manifest hypophosphataemia and this means a low serum ..... .

Phosphate.

Treatment of vitamin resistant rickets, otherwise known as chronic phosphate diabetes, is to give low doses of .... and ..... orally.

Vitamin D; Phosphate.

The administration of Vitamin D does correct the bone changes, but what does it do to the serum phosphate?

Nothing. It does not restore the serum phosphate to normal level.

CHAPTER 33

OSTEOMYELITIS – ACUTE AND CHRONIC

* What is the difference between osteomyelitis and osteitis?

For practical purposes, none. Osteomyelitis implies infection of the bone marrow as well as the bone.

* Is this condition commoner in children or adults?

Children.

* Why is early diagnosis essential?

Because early treatment can avoid development of a chronic osteomyelitis and deformity of bones.

* Name two organisms that commonly cause osteomyelitis in children.

1. Staphylococcus Aureus.
2. Streptococcus.

* The development of the bone infection is usually preceded by a minor ..... to the bone.

Injury.

Pathology

* How do the organisms reach to the bone?

By the blood stream.

* This type of osteomyelitis is called ..... osteomyelitis.

Haematogenous.

* How else may germs set up infection in the bone?

Through an open wound as in a compound fracture.

* With haematogenous osteomyelitis, the infection begins in the ..... of a long bone.

Metaphysis.

Why there? Give two reasons.

1. Increased blood flow to the growing end.
2. Delicate vessels easily injured causing haematoma.

* Where is the metaphysis?

Adjacent to the epiphyseal line, on the shaft side of it.

* When the infection is under way, ... is formed and this soon finds itself at the surface of the bone where it forms a ..... abscess.

Pus.

Sub-periosteal.

How does pus reach the surface from the medulla?

Along Volkmann canals.

* As the abscess expands, it may burst into the ....

Soft tissue.

* If unchecked, an infected clot or thrombus cuts off the blood supply to a part of the bone giving rise to ....

Sequestrum formation.

* The sequestrum is, in effect, a piece of ..... bone.

Dead.

* New bone is laid down under the stripped up periosteum and this new bone is called ..... . Involucrum.

* What prevents the infection spreading into the joint? The epiphyseal cartilage plate.

* If the metaphysis is inside the joint, then septic arthritis readily ..... . Follows.

* Name three metaphyses that are inside the joint.
  1. Upper humerus.
  2. All metaphyses at the elbow.
  3. Upper and lower metaphyses of the femur.

* Does the adjacent joint sometimes swell when no infection is present? Yes, and this is called sympathetic effusion.

* Acute osteomyelitis must be treated early in order to prevent it becoming ..... . Chronic.

* When sequestrum formation has taken place, it may give rise to a .... Discharging sinus.

* Name the other type of osteomyelitis other than haematogenous. Osteomyelitis following compound fracture.

* In compound fractures, how do the organisms enter the bone? Through the open wound.

Clinical Features of Haematogenous Osteomyelitis

* This condition is commonest in ..... and in particular, in ..... . Children.
  Boys.

* Name the bones most commonly affected.
  1. Tibia.
  2. Femur.
  3. Humerus.

* As one would expect, the main symptom is? A child complains of pain at infection site.

* There may be a history of ..... or .... Boils, minor injury.

Physical Examination

* Looking at the patient as a whole, he looks ..... and the thermometer shows a .... Sick; Temperature elevation.

* On assessing the involved part, the examination is divided into four parts. What are they?
  1. Inspection.
  2. Palpation.
  3. Move.
  4. X-ray.

* What do we find on inspection?
  1. The skin may be indurated.
  2. The skin may be red.
  3. The adjacent joint may manifest an effusion.

* What do we find on palpation?
  1. The skin is warm.
  2. Of greater importance, there is exquisite localised tenderness directly over the involved metaphysis.
  3. At a later stage, a fluctuant abscess may be present.

* What is observed on moving the joint?

The movement of the joint is slightly restricted and this distinguishes it from septic arthritis in which the joint movements are grossly restricted and painful.

* What about the radiographs?

In the early stages, these are normal.

* How long after the onset of osteomyelitis would one expect radiographic changes?

Two or three weeks.

* Name two outstanding features on the radiograph in a case of osteomyelitis.

1. Diffuse rarefaction of the metaphyseal area.
2. New bone outlining the raised periosteum.

* Name three changes that can be seen in the blood picture in the case of acute osteomyelitis.

1. Blood culture, positive.
2. Polymorphonuclear leucocytosis.
3. E.S.R. is raised.

The bone scan shows ....

Increased uptake (hot spots).

Before or after X-ray changes?

Before.

* In osteomyelitis secondary to compound fracture the ..... fails to settle after the primary treatment of the wound.

Temperature.

* The wound eventually produces a ..... .

Discharge.

* Which would be the most painful? Acute osteomyelitis that is secondary to a blood borne infection or osteomyelitis secondary to a compound fracture?

The osteomyelitis due to blood borne infection. Haematogenous osteomyelitis is associated with intense pain, whereas compound fracture osteomyelitis is not, as there is already a track for pus to escape.

* With regard to differential diagnosis, acute osteomyelitis must be distinguished from ....

Pyogenic arthritis.

* Give three ways of distinguishing these two conditions.

1. In osteomyelitis, the tenderness is directly over the infected part of the bone and not the adjacent joint.
2. In osteomyelitis, there is a fair range of joint movement maintained.
3. Although in osteomyelitis the joint may be full of fluid, the fluid does not contain pus (this may be confirmed by aspiration).

* When it comes to treating acute osteomyelitis, what must be done before the antibiotics are commenced?

Identify the organism either from drill hole or blood stream.

Complications

* In acute osteomyelitis, the bacteria may stay where they are in the bone indefinitely giving rise to ....

Chronic osteomyelitis.

* Or the bacteria may pass in three directions:

1. Into the joint nearby causing suppurative arthritis.
2. Into the blood stream causing septicaemia, or

3. Involve the epiphyseal cartilage giving rise to retardation of growth of the bone length.

Treatment of Haematogenous Osteomyelitis

* Efficient treatment must be begun at the ..... possible moment.

Earliest.

..... rest is essential.

Bed.

* Name the two antibiotics that should be used systemically even before the organism has been detected and tested for sensitivity. That is, while awaiting the results of blood or pus culture.

Cloxacillin and Penicillin.

* Another possible antibiotic combination would be ..... and ....

Erythromycin; Fusidic Acid.

* These combined antibiotics are used until the .... has been identified and the ..... to which it is most sensitive administered.

Causative organism; Antibiotic.

* For how long should the appropriate antibiotic be given?

For at least four weeks, even if recovery is rapid.

Local Treatment

* Some surgeons feel that antibiotics alone will cure the condition. Most surgeons, however, feel that it is safer to rely on ..... .

Surgery.

* Incising the skin and drilling the bone over the maximum point of tenderness achieves four advantages. What are they?

1. The release of pus.
2. The relief of pain.
3. Reduces the risk of necrosis, e.g. sequestrum formation.
4. Allows identification and sensitivity of the organism.

* One or two drill holes in the bone after the skin has been incised will improve ..... .

Drainage.

* Following drainage, the skin is closed or left open?

Closed.

* Following this operation, the limb is rested in a ..... .

Splint.

The pain of osteomyelitis is very ..... thus requiring ....

Intense.
Adequate analgesia.

Osteomyelitis Complicating Open Fractures

* The treatment is to obtain free ..... through the wound.

Drainage.

* If necessary, the wound can be ..... in order to facilitate drainage.

Enlarged.

* Needless to say, with osteomyelitis complicating open fracture, the appropriate ..... must be used.

Antibiotics.

* Any dead pieces of bone should be ..... .

Removed.

* Chronic osteomyelitis is nearly always a sequel to ....

Acute osteomyelitis.

* Very occasionally the infection may appear as ..... from the beginning.

Chronic.

Chronic Osteomyelitis

* The commonest causative organism is ....

Staphylococcus Aureus.

* Name three other possible causating organisms.

1. Streptococci.
2. Pneumococci.
3. Typhoid bacilli.

Pathology

* Is the condition commoner in long bones or short bones?

Long bones.

* Does chronic osteomyelitis involve one end of the bone or the whole length?

Both — can be at one end or involve the whole length.

* The bone is ..... and ..... than normal.

Thickened; Denser.

* There is a honeycombed appearance which is associated with areas of ..... and ....

Granulation; Fibrous tissue.

* The outstanding features of chronic osteomyelitis, however, are the formation inside the bony cavities of ..... .

Sequestra.

* The other outstanding feature of chronic osteomyelitis is the formation of a .... that leads to the skin surface.

Sinus track.

The usual story is that the sinus tends to heal and then .... recurrently.

Breaks down.

* If a sequestrum is present, the sinus rarely ..... .

Heals.

Clinical Features

* As the pathology tells us, the main symptoms are that of a purulent ..... from a ..... over the affected bone.

Discharge; Sinus.

* Is pain always a feature?

No, it may be intermittent.

* Is the discharge of pus continuous?

No, it is intermittent.

* When the sinus has been quiet and non-discharging for a time and then breaks down giving rise to pyrexia and local pain, this recurrence is called .... or ..... .

Flare up; Flare.

Physical Examination

* When we examine the part, the routine used is divided into four parts. What are they?

1. Inspection.
2. Palpation.
3. Move.
4. X-ray.

* What do we observe on inspection of the area?

A thickened bone, a reddish skin and perhaps a discharging sinus.

* What do we feel on palpation?

Increased temperature of the skin adjacent to the sinus plus tenderness.

* What do we find with movement?

Nothing.

* What about the radiographs?

They show four features.

* What are they?

1. Thickened bone.
2. Areas of sclerosis.
3. Sequestrum formation.
4. Cavity formation.

* Name one complication of chronic osteomyelitis that can also be a feature of any chronic infection that produces pus over a long period of time.

Amyloid Disease.

Treatment

* Firstly, the acute flare up is treated with ..... and ..... .

Rest.
Antibiotics.

* Infected dead bone, known as sequestra, have to be ..... .

Removed.

* Abscess cavities have to be adequately ..... .

Drained.

* Name two other ways of dealing with a cavity in the bone.

1. Sometimes it can be obliterated with a flap of muscle.
2. Occasionally it can be lined with a split skin graft.

Brodie's Abscess — A Chronic Bone Abscess

* What is the difference between Brodie's abscess and any other type of chronic osteomyelitis?

Brodie's abscess arises insidiously without a preceding acute attack.

* Where is the Brodie's Abscess usually located?

In the metaphysis of a bone.

* What is the main symptom?

A boring pain at the site of the Brodie's Abscess.

* What is the typical radiographic appearance?

It appears as a circular or oval cavity surrounded by a zone of dense white sclerotic bone — the rest of the bone being normal.

The treatment of the Brodie's Abscess is to decorticate the ..... and where possible to obliterate the dead space inside the cavity by filling it with a ....

Cavity.

Muscle flap.

149

CHAPTER 34

PYOGENIC ARTHRITIS

What are the other two names for pyogenic arthritis?

Infective arthritis and septic arthritis.

Name four organisms that can cause pyogenic arthritis.

1. Staphylococcus Aureus.
2. Streptococcus.
3. Pneumococcus.
4. Gonococcus.

* How does the organism reach the joint? Give three routes.

1. Through the blood stream (haematogenous infection).
2. Through penetrating wound.
3. By extension of adjacent focus of osteomyelitis.

Name four joints in which the metaphysis is wholly or partly within the joint cavity.

1. Upper humeral metaphysis.
2. Metaphyses at the elbow.
3. Upper metaphysis of femur.
4. Lower metaphysis of femur.

What is the significance of the position of the metaphysis so far as pyogenic arthritis is concerned?

In osteomyelitis, the metaphysis is the site of infection and if the metaphysis is in the joint, then pyogenic arthritis takes place very easily.

The infection causes a gathering of .... in the joint.

Infected fluid.

* There are two possible outcomes to pyogenic arthritis. What are they?

1. Complete resolution with normal function.
2. Total destruction of the joint and fibrous or bony ankylosis.

Clinical Features

* Name two symptoms of pyogenic arthritis pertaining to the joint.

1. Swelling of the joint.
2. Pain.

Name two clinical features pertaining to the general bodily function.

1. Constitutional illness and nausea.
2. Pyrexia.

* Name the four features of the examination of a joint.

1. Inspection.
2. Palpation.
3. Move.
4. X-ray.

* What two features are seen on inspection?

A redness and swelling of the joint.

* What features are discovered on palpation?

Increased temperature of the skin adjacent to the joint plus fluctuation.

* What about movements of the joint?

All are restricted.

* What two features might be found on the radiograph?

1. A normal radiograph is seen in the early stages.
2. Later loss of cartilage and destruction of bone.

* Name three investigations you would arrange to clinch the diagnosis of pyogenic arthritis.

1. Aspirated joint fluid contains causative organisms.
2. Raised E.S.R.
3. Raised white cell count (polymorphs).

* How does one distinguish pyogenic arthritis from osteomyelitis?

With osteomyelitis, there is a well-defined tender area adjacent to the joint in the metaphysis. In pyogenic arthritis, the joint movements are more severely restricted than in osteomyelitis.

Name three other types of arthritis that must be distinguished from pyogenic arthritis.

1. Tuberculous arthritis (very rare nowadays).
2. Gouty arthritis.
3. Haemophilic arthritis. Usually there is a history of haemophilia.

The prognosis is such that the joint does one of two things.

1. Returns completely to normal if treatment is prompt.
2. It may be totally destroyed giving rise to a fibrous or bony ankylosis.

Treatment

* Why is early treatment essential?

To prevent destruction of the joint.

Give six features of local treatment.

1. Rest joint in plaster splint.
2. Aspirate fluid from the joint.
3. Replace this with penicillin.
4. Send aspirated fluid to Bacteriology Department to assess nature of organism and its sensitivity.
5. Aspirate joint and replace with appropriate antibiotic daily.
6. When temperature and swelling have subsided, start mobilising patient out of bed.

General treatment consists of .... and ....

1. Bed Rest.
2. Administration of intravenous or oral antibiotics to which the organism has been proved sensitive.

Subsequent Treatment

If the articular cartilage is **not** injured, how would you proceed?

Go for movement with gentle gradual exercises. Weight bearing with a splint initially then the splint is discarded.

If articular cartilage is destroyed, what then?

Splint joint in optimum position until ankylosis is established, then commence weight bearing.

CHAPTER 35

TUMOURS OF BONE

Bone tumours are classified into three groups. What are they?

1. Benign.
2. Primary malignant.
3. Secondary malignant.

* What is the other name for a secondary tumour?

Metastatic tumour.

How many benign tumours are there?

Four.

How many malignant tumours are there?

Six.

Benign Tumours of Bone

It is easy to work out the benign tumours of bone because bone is made up of bone cells and cartilage cells.

* The tumours arising from bone cells are called ..... .

Osteomas.

* The tumours arising from cartilage cells are called ..... .

Chondromas.

* The tumours arising from both of these elements would naturally be called ..... .

Osteochondromas.

Name two types of osteoma.

Ivory osteoma and spongy or cancellous osteoma.

Name two bones from which it might arise.

1. The skull.
2. Any long bone.

Name two ways of treating an osteoma.

1. Either do nothing since it is harmless, or
2. Excise it.

Chondroma

Chondromas either grow towards the centre of the bone or grow outwards. The chondroma that grows outwards from a bone is called an ..... .

Ecchondroma.

The chondroma that grows within a bone is called an ..... .

Enchondroma.

Both these types of chondroma appear commonly in ..... or ..... .

Hands; feet.

Since the expanding tumour thins out the cortex, the tumour often presents with a ....

Pathological fracture.

Multiple enchondromata arising in several bones in children constitute a condition called ..... disease.

Ollier's.

In this condition of Ollier's disease, why does the child have deformities and shortening of the bone?

Because enchondromata involve the epiphyseal cartilages thus disrupting normal bone growth.

Do chondromata ever become malignant?

Yes, rarely. They turn inro chondrosarcomas.

So these chondrosarcomas occur in major bones or small bones of the feet?

Usually in major bones.

Treatment of Chondromata

Give two ways of treating chondromata.

1. Do nothing.
2. Remove it if it is unsightly or causing trouble.

Osteochondroma

This is the ..... benign tumour of bone.

Commonest.

This tumour is well known because it is composed of both ..... and ..... .

Bone; cartilage.

The cartilage element of the tumour arises from ....

Epiphyseal cartilage.

The tumour grows outwards from the bone like a ..... .

Mushroom.

The stalk and part of the head of the mushroom are composed of ..... .

Bone.

The very top of the head of the mushroom is capped by ..... .

Cartilage.

Usually the osteochondroma is single but there is a condition in which there are multiple tumours. Name this condition.

Diaphyseal aclasis, a familial disorder.

What is the commonest site for an osteochondroma?

Lower femur.

The radiographs of the hard lump of which the patient complains, show a .... etc.

Mushroom shaped swelling growing away from the knee joint, going upwards and outwards.

Is the cartilage cap seen on the radiograph?

No, cartilage does not show on radiographs.

In 1% of cases what happens to the cartilage cap?

Changes to chondrosarcoma.

What is the treatment for osteochondroma?

When necessary, the tumour should be excised.

Osteoid Osteoma

Define osteoid osteoma.

A benign tumour of bone consisting of a radio-translucent peripheral area (NIDUS) surrounding a central area of newly formed bone.

What is the usual size?

1 cm or less — round or oval.

What surrounds the lesion?

Dense bone.

Name two common sites.	1. Femur.
	2. Tibia.
Give the main symptom.	Pain.
Differential diagnosis – give three.	1. Brodie's abscess (biopsy it).
	2. Ewing's tumour.
	3. Chronic periostitis.
Give one special diagnostic test.	Bone scan.
Treatment – give one.	Excision is curative.

Osteoclastoma

The last of the benign tumours is the giant cell tumour, otherwise known as	Osteoclastoma.
Is it really benign?	No.
What is the fate of one third of them?	They are locally invasive.
What is the fate of another third?	They metastasize.
This benign tumour exhibits two qualities, usually associated with malignant tumours. What are they?	1. It tends to recur after local removal.
	2. Sometimes it metastasizes through the blood stream.
What is the common age group for the osteoclastoma?	Young adults.

Pathology of Giant Cell Tumour or Osteoclastoma

Give the four common sites for an osteoclastoma.	1. Lower end of femur.
	2. Upper end of tibia.
	3. Lower end of radius.
	4. Upper end of humerus.
The giant cell tumour or osteoclastoma begins in that part of the bone that used to be the	Metaphyseal Region.
It then crosses a boundary. Which boundary?	Epiphyseal cartilage.
In so doing, it reaches the ..... of the bone.	End.
Sometimes it reaches almost to the joint	Surface.
The word osteoclast implies removal of bone just as osteoblast implies ..... of bone.	Deposition.
So the osteoclastoma destroys the bone substance but the periosteum lays down new bone thus giving rise to an expanded	End.
Since the bone is very weak, this tumour frequently presents with a .... in 10-15% of cases.	Pathological fracture.
When a giant cell tumour is seen histologically under the microscope, what is the typical cell to be seen?	Giant cell.

154

How many nuclei might be in a single giant cell?

Up to fifty.

Do the giant cells resemble the osteoclasts closely?

No.

Is the osteoclastoma therefore a good name for this tumour?

No. It is better known as a giant cell tumour.

When this tumour is malignant, it metastasizes mainly to ....

The lungs.

Clinical Features

As one would expect with a large expanding tumour at the end of a bone, the two outstanding symptoms are ..... and ..... .

Swelling; Pain.

Occasionally the tumour presents as a ..... fracture.

Pathological.

Radiographs show three features. What are they?

1. Destruction of bone substance.
2. Expansion of the cortex.
3. "Soap bubble" appearance.

Treatment of Giant Cell Tumour

The three weapons we have in the treatment of giant cell tumour are:

1. Total excision.
2. Curettage.
3. Radiotherapy.

If the affected bone is one that we can do without such as the ..... and ....., excision of part or whole of the bone is recommended to ensure complete removal of the tumour.

Clavicle; Fibula.

If the bone is a vital one such as the femur, the best course is probably wide local ..... even if this means replacing the adjacent joint with ..... or by joint ..... .

Excision.
A prosthesis.
Fusion.

Curettage followed by packing with bone grafts was complicated by a high rate of ..... .

Recurrence.

This was frequently followed by ..... .

Amputation.

Radiotherapy may do two things. What are they?

1. Produce permanent cure.
2. Induce malignant change.

Radiotherapy then is confined to tumours at sites that are ..... to surgery.

Inaccessible.

Malignant Tumours

When classifying tumours of bone, we can think along the lines that bone is made up of bone cells, cartilage cells and fibrous tissue, so three tumours from that area would constitute the following.

1. Osteosarcoma.
2. Chondrosarcoma.
3. Fibrosarcoma.

Bone also has a medullary cavity whose cells produce some of the cells of the blood stream and so one could expect tumours arising from that part. Name two.

1. Multiple myeloma.
2. Leukemia.

What is another name for a plasmacytoma?

Myeloma.

Tumours may also arrive at a bone from other parts of the body and these are known as ....

Metastatic Tumours.

The final malignant tumour to be discussed is obscure in origin and closely resembles a metastatic tumour. What is its name?

Ewing's tumour.

Secondary (Metastatic) Tumours in Bone

Which are the commoner malignant tumours of bone, primary or secondary?

Secondary.

Most primary malignant bone tumours occur in ..... or ....

Children; Young adults.

Secondary tumours generally occur in ..... life.

Later.

Tumours that commonly spread to bone are carcinomas from two midline structures and three other paired structures. What are they?

Prostate and thyroid glands. Lung, breast and kidneys.

The only significance of whether they are paired or midline is to aid your memory.

This is a frequently asked question so draw a diagram many times so it is clear in the mind that carcinomas of the prostate, thyroid, breast, lung and kidneys spread or metastasize to ..... .

Bone.

Metastases occur most commonly in the parts of the skeleton that contain vascular marrow. What are they?

1. Vertebral bodies.
2. Ribs.
3. Pelvis.
4. Upper end of femur.
5. Upper end of humerus.

Since the tumour destroys and replaces bone structure, it frequently presents with a pathological ..... .

Fracture.

The two main presenting symptoms with a secondary bone tumour are:

1. Pain at site of secondary.
2. Pathological fracture.

Is the primary tumour readily demonstrated in most cases?

Yes.

The radiographic examination is most important. In most cases with secondaries in bone, the radiograph shows a clear, circumscribed area of trans ..... .

Radiance.

In most cases then, there is no attempt at further bone formation around the metastatic deposit. Give one exception to this rule where marked sclerosis does take place.

Secondary deposits from prostatic carcinoma.

What is the reason for the increased density?

Large quantities of phosphatase in the cells.

What investigation will allow early detection of asymptomatic metastatic deposits?

The bone scan.

A bone seeking substance is given by intravenous injection and this is then picked up with the aid of a ..... counter.

Geiger.

From your knowledge of bone structure, what intravenous isotope would probably be used to be a bone seeker?

A phosphorus-containing one such as technetium with diphosphonate.

This isotope known fully as 99M technetium with diphosphonate is conveyed rapidly to the bone and the emitted rays are charted by means of a gamma ..... .

Camera.

Since the bone seeking isotope gets to the bone by the blood stream, one would expect an in-increased concentration of the bone seeking isotope in a situation where there is ..... of the bone.

Hyperaemia.

In the case of prostatic metastases, there is one specific blood test that is helpful. What is it?

In this condition, the acid phosphatase in the blood is usually increased above the normal 1-3 King Armstrong units per 100 mls.

What is the normal value in King Armstrong units per 100 mls.?

1 to 3 King Armstrong units.

Is it acid phosphatase or alkaline phosphatase that is raised in patients with prostatic metastases?

Acid phosphatase is raised above the normal 1 to 3 K.A. units.

Treatment

In conditions where there is a secondary bone deposit from carcinoma of the thyroid, what radioactive substance may be of use?

Radioactive iodine.

Since tumours of the breast are said to be hormone dependent, what therapy could be of value in dealing with tumours of the breast?

Tomoxafin, an antioestrogen compound.

Likewise, wirh prostatic secondaries, name a hormone that might be of value in treatment.

Stilboestrol.

Name one operation that inhibits hormone production that might be of value in carcinoma of breast or prostate.

Adrenalectomy.

Name another that may help with prostatic tumour.

Orchidectomy (excision of testes).

What about the management of the pathological fracture from the point of view of the patient's comfort — what two procedures could be helpful?

The fracture can be splinted or internally fixated, using acrylic cement if need be.

What about the relief of pain in these conditions? How is this achieved?

Analgesics and sedatives may be given plus radiotherapy.

Ewing's Tumour (Endothelial Sarcoma of Bone)

Tumours discussed above have arisen from bone cells or cartilage cells or fibrous tissue of bone but this tumour, namely Ewing's tumour, probably arises from bone ..... .

Marrow.

Is Ewing's tumour rare or common?

Rare.

Is Ewing's tumour relatively benign or malignant?

It is highly malignant.

Pathology

The tumours mentioned above from bone and cartilage and fibrous tissue etc., usually arise at the end of long bones but the Ewing's tumour is usually situated in the middle of which bones? Give three.

In the shaft of:
1. Femur or
2. Tibia or
3. Humerus.

As it expands from the bone marrow, the soft vascular tumour destroys the ....

Bone; Substance.

Which vegetable does Ewing's tumour remind you of?

The onion.

The reason for this is that as the periosteum is pushed outwards, new bone is formed in successive layers giving the appearance of the onion peel. So the onion peel effect reminds you of ....

Ewing's tumour.

What is the histological appearance of the Ewing's tumour?

Small, round cells in large sheets.

Whence do the metastases spread?

Via the blood stream to the lungs and sometimes to other bones.

What about the prognosis of Ewing's tumour?

Nearly always fatal due to pulmonary metastases.

Clinical Features of Ewing's Tumour

Is this tumour more common in children or adults? Give the age group.

Children, i.e. 10-20 years.

Whereas with other malignant tumours mentioned above we have a lump or swelling and pain at the end of the long bone, with Ewing's tumour the pain and swelling is usually about the ..... of the shaft.

Middle.

Give two symptoms.	1. Throbbing pain. 2. Limp.
When feeling this tumour, the skin is ..... than normal owing to the vascularity of the tumour.	Warmer.
What vegetable does the radiograph remind you of and why?	The onion because the radiographs show concentric layers like an onion peel in the sub-perio-steum.
What other radiographs should be taken when this condition is suspected?	Lung fields might reveal metastases.

Diagnosis

As with osteosarcoma, this condition has to be distinguished from acute inflammatory and chronic inflammatory lesions as well as other tumours. What are these inflammatory conditions and name three other tumours.	1. Sub-acute osteomyelitis and
	2. Syphilitic osteomyelitis.
	3. Other tumours such as:
	    osteosarcoma,
	    fibrosarcoma,
	    chondrosarcoma.

There is a particular secondary bone tumour that might simulate Ewing's tumour. Name it.	Suprarenal neuroblastoma.
How is the diagnosis of Ewing's tumour finally clinched?	By biopsy.

Treatment of Ewing's Tumour

As one could expect, there are three possibilities. What are they?	1. Amputation. 2. Chemotherapy. 3. Radiotherapy. Chemotherapy now gives better results than radiotherapy.
Radiotherapy would avoid the ..... trauma of an amputation in a young person.	Psychological.

Osteosarcoma

What is the other name for osteosarcoma?	Osteogenic sarcoma.
What is the commonest age group for this tumour?	Childhood or early adult life, i.e. 10-20 years.
When it occurs in later life, it is usually a complication of another common bone disease. What is it?	Paget's disease.

Pathology

From which cells does this tumour arise?	Primitive bone forming cells.
Describe the histopath.	Spindle cells with many mitoses.
In what part of which bones is it commonly seen?	Lower end of femur, upper end of tibia, upper end of humerus.

From what part of the bone of the child does the tumour arise?

The metaphysis.

Does it usually cross the epiphyseal cartilage and enter the epiphysis?

No.

Name three types of tissue that may be seen in this tumour.

1. Fibrous tissue.
2. Cartilage or
3. Myxomatous tissue.

Name the two varieties of bone cells also seen.

1. Osteoblasts.
2. Osteoclasts.

In all these tumours, however, ... tissue is always found.

Osteoid.

What is Codman's triangle?

The angle between the elevated periosteum and the shaft and is the smallest angle of the triangle.

How does the tumour metastasize?

By the blood stream.

Whence do they travel? Give two.

To the lungs and to other bones.

Clinical Features

Give the three main clinical features of this tumour.

1. Local pain near the joint.
2. Swelling near the joint.
3. Hard bony thickening is felt at the end of the long bone. If osteoclasts predominate, the tumour may be soft.

Give two radiographic features.

1. The raised periosteum forms one side of a triangle with the cortex of the bone and this triangle is called Codman's triangle.
2. The second feature is the sun-ray appearance of the tumour and this is produced by radiating spicules of new bone seen within the tumour.

What might a chest radiograph reveal?

Pulmonary metastases.

Diagnosis

A swelling at the end of a long bone in a child or young adult may be due to many other lesions. Name seven.

1. Sub-acute osteomyelitis.
2. Syphilis of bone.
3. Chondrosarcoma.
4. Fibrosarcoma.
5. Giant cell tumour.
6. Ewing's tumour.
7. Metastatic tumour.

How would one clinch the diagnosis?

Biopsy and histological examination.

What is the mortality rate with osteosarcoma?

About 65% to 85% mortality rate (even after amputation) is the usual finding.

Treatment of Osteosarcoma

Give three methods of treating this highly malignant tumour.

1. Amputation immediately after diagnosis by biopsy.
2. High voltage radiotherapy to sterilize tumour cells, followed by amputation in six months if chest X-ray fails to reveal metastases.
3. A preliminary amputation followed by the modern cytotoxic drugs seems to be a hopeful way of controlling metastases for a long time.

What are the cytotoxic drugs?

1. Oncovin.
2. Methotrexate.
3. Doxorubicin.

Chondrosarcoma of Bone

From which cells are these tumours derived?

From cartilage cells.

From a pathological point of view, what are the two types?

1. Central chondrosarcoma in the interior of the bone.
2. Peripheral chondrosarcoma on the surface.

Where does one find a central chondrosarcoma? Give three locations.

1. The femur.
2. The tibia.
3. The humerus.

Give the name of a benign tumour that may give rise to a chondrosarcoma of the central type.

Enchondroma may give rise to a chondrosarcoma.

A peripheral chondrosarcoma may arise from which benign tumour?

From an osteochondroma.

What are the main histological findings of a chondrosarcoma?

Cartilage cells are seen with the occasional double nuclei.

Clinical Features

What is the commonest age group?

Middle age, i.e. 35-55.

What are the two main complaints with which the patient presents?

1. Pain at site of lesion.
2. Swelling at site of lesion.

Radiographically the central chondrosarcoma behaves in what fashion?

It may burst through the cortex as it expands outwards.

A peripheral chondrosarcoma on the other hand, tends to grow in which direction?

Outwards from the surface of the bone.

How malignant is the chondrosarcoma?

It is a slow growing tumour and does not metastasize early.

How is it best treated?

Early amputation well removed from the tumour area gives a reasonable prospect of cure; in conjunction with chemotherapy.

Fibrosarcoma

Is this common or rare?

Very rare.

Which is the commonest age group?	Young adults.
Which are the commonest bones? Give two.	1. The femur.
	2. The tibia.
The main histological feature is the presence of ..... cells.	Fibroblast.
The main radiographic finding is that of an ..... lesion.	Osteolytic.
What is the prognosis like?	It is poor but not as unfavourable as osteosarcoma.
Which is the best form of treatment?	Wide local excision.
Does it respond to irradiation?	No.

Multiple Myeloma

Like Ewing's tumour, the myeloma arises from	Bone marrow.
Give two other names for multiple myeloma.	1. Myelomatosis.
	2. Plasmacytoma.
Is the myeloma commoner in children or adults?	It is usually seen in adults.
So of all the tumours of bone that we have discussed up to date, most are seen in young people, but in adults, we see the condition of	Multiple myeloma.
What is the prognosis in myelomatosis?	Almost uniformly fatal.

Pathology

Which is the most likely cell that produces myelomatosis?	The plasma cell.
By the time this condition is diagnosed, it has usually spread to many parts of the skeleton and in particular, to that part of the marrow known as the ..... marrow.	Red.
So the red marrow is usually the site of multiple tumour foci in this condition of	Myelomatosis.
The lesions of myelomatosis are mainly small and	Circumscribed.
The extraordinary and sinister feature of the myeloma is that the tumour replaces the bone and there is no attempt at new bone formation so ..... fracture is very common.	Pathological.
Since the tumour is seen mainly in ..... marrow, a common site for it is in the ..... column.	Red. Vertebral.
The red marrow of the vertebral bodies is invaded and weakened, giving rise to pathological ..... of the bone.	Fractures.

Fractures of the spine may, of course, cause compression of the .... giving rise to ..... .

Spinal cord; Paraplegia.

What is paraplegia?

Paralysis of motor and sensory function from about the waist level downwards.

Histologically, the tumour consists of cells that resemble the cells of origin. What are the cells of origin?

Plasma cells.

The only difference from plasma cells seen in this tumour is that they are ..... than normal.

Larger.

Furthermore, they are less ..... .

Uniform.

Clinical Features of Myelomatosis

Is the patient more often older or younger than middle age?

Older. Past middle age.

There is general ill ..... with ..... at one or more tumour sites.

Health; Pain.

On examination, the patient looks tired and due to malfunction of red blood cell formation, is ..... .

Pale.

There is often local ..... over the affected bones, but quite often the condition presents with a pathological ..... .

Tenderness.

Fracture.

Radiographs show multiple areas of ....

Trans radiance.

Translucence means "light penetrates the part" and so trans radiance means that ..... penetrate the part.

X-rays.

The reason for the trans radiance is that the tumour destroys the ..... and no further bone ..... takes place.

Bone
Formation.

The multiple areas of trans radiance occur especially in bones containing red marrow and they are:

1. Ribs.
2. Vertebral bodies.
3. Pelvic bones.
4. Skull.
5. Proximal end of femur.
6. Proximal end of humerus.

What is the usual cause of death?

Renal failure.

Investigations

What two abnormalities are found in the blood stream in myelomatosis?

1. Normochromic normocytic anaemia.
2. E.S.R. raised.
   (E = erythrocyte
   (S = sedimentation
   (R = rate).

With myelomatosis, what may be found in the urine?

Bence Jones proteins are present in more than half the cases.

When myelomatosis is suspected, then examine the urine for ....

Bence Jones proteins.

In what percentage do you expect to find Bence Jones proteins?

More than fifty percent.

What investigation of serum protein is likely to give a positive result?

Serum electrophoretogram may show a peak at an abnormal point identifying the abnormal protein being produced.

Since the tumour arises from plasma cells, a marrow biopsy would show a profusion of ..... cells.

Plasma.

The diagnosis of myelomatosis is clinched by ..... biopsy.

Marrow.

From what part of the body does one obtain a marrow biopsy?

From the marrow of iliac crest or from the sternum.

What is the prognosis with myelomatosis?

Usually fatal, although life can be prolonged for many years.

Treatment

If you didn't know the treatment, you could guess at two methods.

1. Radiotherapy for tumour foci.
2. Cytotoxic drugs such as Cyclophosphamide or Melphalan.

Leukaemia and Hodgkin's Disease

Do you think that bone changes can take place sometimes with leukaemia and Hodgkin's disease. Yes or No?

Yes.

As you might guess, the changes are similar to those of a bone metastasis and these changes in leukaemias are due to infiltration of the bone by those cells that proliferate in leukaemia. What are those cells?

White cells.

Proliferation of white cells infiltrating the bone is commonly seen in adults or children. Which?

Children.

So the two changes on the X-ray seen in leukaemia are ..... and ....

Rarefaction; sub-periosteal new bone formation.

In what part of the bone would rarefaction and sub-periosteal new bone formation take place and be seen radiologically in children with leukaemia?

In the metaphysis region of certain bones.

In what bones would one see rarefaction and sub-periosteal new bone formation in children with leukaemia?

In the metaphysis of the femur or humerus or in the spine or pelvis.

Leukemia may occasionally be present with widespread ..... of the skeleton.

Rarefaction.

With regard to Hodgkin's disease, ... lesions in proximal limb bones are frequently seen.

Osteolytic.

164

As with secondary or metastatic deposits from many primary sites, the osteolytic lesion indicates destruction of bone without any attempt at bone ..... .

Replacement.

Aneurysmal Bone Cyst

Define aneurysmal bone cyst.

A lesion that simulates a tumour and featuring cavities filled with blood.

Give two common sites.

1. Spine (vertebral body).
2. Metaphysis of long bones.

It expands thus destroying the ..... .

Cortex.

Give two radiographic features.

1. Area of rarefaction.
2. Eccentrically placed.

The aneurysmal bone cyst has to be distinguished from ....

Giant cell tumour.

What is the difference?

Giant cell tumour extends to the articular surface.
Aneurysmal bone cyst stays at metaphysis.

How is it treated?

Curettage and packing with bone chips.

CHAPTER 36

RHEUMATOID ARTHRITIS

* Define rheumatoid arthritis.

Rheumatoid arthritis is a non-infective systemic disease of obscure origin causing pain, swelling and deformity of joints associated with chronic inflammation in the synovia of both joints and tendons.

* Which bacteria are involved with rheumatoid arthritis?

None. Rheumatoid arthritis is a chronic non-bacterial inflammation of the joints.

* Is it usually one joint involved or more than one?

Almost always more than one (polyarthritis).

Name four medical conditions that show similar joint changes.

1. Still's disease.
2. Reiter's syndrome.
3. Psoriasis.
4. Lupus erythematosus.

* What is the cause of rheumatoid arthritis?

Not known, possibly a virus associated with abnormal immune response.

* What two parts of the joint are involved in pathology of rheumatoid arthritis?

1. The synovial membrane.
2. The articular cartilage.

* What happens to the synovial membrane in rheumatoid arthritis?

Chronic inflammation thickens the membrane.

* What happens to the articular cartilage in rheumatoid arthritis?

It becomes softened and eroded.

Clinical Features

* What is the age range?

Twenty-forty years.

* What is the incidence?

3% of population suffer R.A.

* Are the central joints or peripheral joints mainly affected with this condition?

Peripheral joints much more common, e.g., joints of hands, wrist, feet, knees and elbows.

What is the sex ratio?

Three times commoner in women.

* What are the early features?

Increasing pain and swelling of several peripheral joints.

What are Apley's four criteria for diagnosis of rheumatoid arthritis?

1. Bilateral polyarthritis.
2. Proximal joints of hands or feet involved.
3. The above present for at least six weeks.
4. Positive rheumatoid factor test.

* How do we examine a joint?

1. Inspection.
2. Palpation.
3. Move.
4. X-ray.

* With rheumatoid arthritis, what do we see on inspection?

Swollen, red and perhaps deformed joints.

* Palpation?

The joint is warm.

* Move?

The range of movement is limited and moving causes pain.

* X-ray findings.

Early — nil. Later — diffuse rarefaction of bones adjacent to the joint due to increased vascularity.
Later joint destruction leading to narrowing of the joint space and erosion of bone ends.

* What is the classical finding on examining the blood?

E.S.R. is raised during the active phase and anti-IgG globulins appear in the serum.

Differential diagnosis from Still's disease, Reiter's syndrome, Lupus erythematosus and psoriasis.

1. Still's disease — confined to children, spleen and lymphatic glands enlarged.
2. Reiter's syndrome — urethritis, arthritis and conjunctivitis and hyperkeratotic eruptions on the skin.
3. Lupus erythematosus shows scaling erythema of face or other parts.
4. Psoriasis — has typical patchy skin lesions.

What is meant by the rheumatoid factors?

Anti-IgG globulins in the serum in 80% of cases.

What is the significance of persistently high titres in rheumatoid factor test?

The persistently high titre means a more serious disease.

In most cases of rheumatoid arthritis there is .... of joint function.

Permanent impairment.

In certain joints — especially the knees, ... is often superimposed upon the burnt-out rheumatoid condition.

Osteoarthritis.

Treatment of Rheumatoid Arthritis

* Is there a specific cure for rheumatoid arthritis?

No.

* Name five drugs that can give some relief for this condition.

1. Butazolidine.
2. Aspirin.
3. Penicillamine.
4. Steroids — i.e. Immuno-suppressive drug.
5. Gold salts.

How do 1. and 2. above work?

They control pain and stiffness and help function but don't arrest the disease.

How do 3., 4. and 5. work?

They have a direct action on the immunopathological process, but have devastating side effects on liver, kidney and haemopoietic system.

* What steroids are used?

Cortisone or prednisone.

* Do they sometimes produce a dramatic effect?

Yes, pain and stiffness may be dramatically relieved.

* Why must we be wary of the steroids?

Very serious side effects may follow prolonged use. Sudden cessation may cause adrenal suppression.

* What are the side effects?

Cushing's disease. Obesity and pathological fractures.

How are these side effects monitored?

With regular blood tests and liver and renal function tests.

Local Treatment of Rheumatoid Arthritis

* When the condition is very early and acute, ... the joint and treat it with ....

Immobilize; Ice packs.

* When it becomes less acute and more moderate, ... the joint.

Exercise.

* Name five methods of physiotherapy that can give relief to the recovering joint.

1. Infra-red radiation.
2. Shortwave diathermy.
3. Hot packs.
4. Wax baths.
5. Hydrotherapy.

Can injections of nitrogen mustard or hydrocortisone into the joints help?

Yes, sometimes.

What effect does synovectomy have?

May arrest disease in that joint.

* In the established disease the fingers manifest ..... deviation.

Ulnar.

Name three operations that can be performed on joints for the pain and stiffness when the disease is burnt out.

1. Joint replacement.
2. Excision arthroplasty (simply excising the bones that constitute the joint).
3. Joint arthrodesis, e.g. stiffening a wrist joint by placing bone graft across the joint that has been decorticated.

When is tendon surgery indicated?

When they rupture thus predisposing to deformity.

CHAPTER 37

BACK PAIN

Give ten common causes of low back pain.

1. Prolapsed intervertebral disc.
2. Osteoarthritis of facet joints.
3. Muscle strain — or ligamentous injury.
4. Spondylolisthesis.
5. Tumour of the spinal column.
6. Ankylosing spondylitis.
7. Tumour of ilium or sacrum.
8. Intrapelvic mass, e.g. tumour of rectum, prostate or uterus.
9. Tumour of the cord or cauda equina.
10. Fracture.

Returning to the prolapsed lumbar intervertebral disc, give two possible causes of this.

1. Injuries.
2. Age — degeneration.

Which is the commonest disc to be affected in the lumbar spine?

L—5. S—1.

Which nerve root would be involved with an L—5. S—1 disc lesion?

First sacral nerve root.

Would involvement of the first sacral nerve root give rise to weakness of dorsi flexion or plantar flexion?

Plantar flexion.

Would the numbness with S—1 malfunction be in the front of the thigh or the sole of the foot?

Mainly sole of foot.

Why is the L—5. S—1 disc the commonest to be affected?

Because (being the lowest disc) it takes maximum weight.

Name the two parts of a lumbar disc.

Annulus fibrosus and nucleus pulposus.

In the process of disc prolapse, how many phases are there?

Three.

In the first phase, a ..... appears in the annulus fibrosus.

Crack.

In the second phase, the .... goes through the crack and touches the posterior longitudinal ligament giving rise to ....

Nucleus pulposus.

Back pain.

With further prolapse of nucleus through the crack in the ....., the nerve ..... is involved giving rise to ..... .

Annulus; Root.
Sciatica.

There are two main symptoms of lumbar disc prolapse, namely low back pain plus or minus sciatica, and the pain or pains are worsened by six factors. What are they?

1. Coughing.
2. Sneezing.
3. Stooping.
4. Lifting.
5. Sitting.
6. Standing.

The pain of a lumbar disc lesion is usually relieved by ..... .

Reclining.

What is the drill when we examine the back?

1. Inspection.
2. Palpation.
3. Move.
4. X-ray.

On looking or inspecting the back, we might see a spine that has two features.

s\B
Tilt (with spasm) or scoliosis.

When palpating the lumbar part tenderness is located either in .... or ....

The midline.
One cm to right or left of the midline.

What are the six movements of the lumbar spine that we test?

1. Flexion.
2. Extension.
3. Tilt right.
4. Tilt left.
5. Rotation to right.
6. Rotation to left.

On examining the lumbar spine, we must of course, examine the lower limbs because the nerves from the spine going into the limbs influence the function of the limb.

* What are the five main features we look for in the lower limbs?

1. Motor power.
2. Sensory.
3. Reflex.
4. Measure — for wasting.
5. Straight leg raising.

* Since with disc prolapse either L—4—5 or L—5. S—1 is the disc usually involved, the motor power we have to test is simply .... for L—5. S—1 and .... for an L—4—5 disc lesion.

Plantar
flexion; Dorsi flexion.

* With an L—4—5 disc lesion, the usual nerve root involved is ..... .

L—5.

* Sensory malfunction with an L—4—5 nerve root would involve the cleft between ..... and ..... toes.

First.
Second.

* Sensory malfunction involving an S—1 dermatome would involve three parts of the foot. What are they?

1. Outer dorsal aspect.
2. Lateral border.
3. Outer plantar aspect.

* Which nerve root is involved mainly with the knee jerk?

L—4.

* Which reflex is involved with the fifth lumbar nerve root?

Hamstring jerk.

* Which nerve root is involved mainly with the ankle jerk?

The S—1 nerve root.

* Why do we measure the thigh and calf musculature?

To see if they are wasted as a result of a motor weakness.

* Why is straight leg raising painful with a prolapsed disc?

Because the nerve root, either L–5 or S–1, is being stretched over the prolapsed disc on straight leg raising.

* Give five methods of conservative treatment for a prolapsed lumbar disc.

1. Enforced bed rest with leg or pelvic traction till symptoms subside.
2. Spinal extension exercises.
3. Plaster jacket or corset.
4. Manipulation of spine.
5. Injection of Depomedrol into either the subarachnoid space or intradiscally.

* Give four indications for surgery for a prolapsed lumbar intervertebral disc.

1. Agonizing uncontrollable pain.
2. Paralysis of part or all of the lower limb.
3. Failed twelve weeks conservative treatment.
4. Impaired bladder or bowel function.

* What operation would be performed for the situation where sciatica is the most pronounced symptom?

Laminectomy and disc excision with decompression of the nerve root throughout its length.

* Which operation would be suitable for the situation where backache predominates?

Spinal fusion.

Where is the defect in spondylolysis?

In the pars interarticularis.

What is the significance of spondylolysis?

It may be a precursor to spondylolisthesis because the defect allows one vertebral body to slide forward on the other.

Definition of Spondylolisthesis

Define spondylolisthesis.

Spondylolisthesis is a condition in which one vertebral body spontaneously slips forwards or backwards upon the vertebral body below it.

Give three possible causes of spondylolisthesis.

1. Defect in the pars interarticularis.
2. Secondary to osteoarthritis of the posterior intervertebral joints.
3. Secondary to congenital malformation of the articular processes.

What are the symptoms of spondylolisthesis? Give two.

1. No symptoms.
2. Chronic backache plus or minus sciatica.

With regard to the signs of spondylolisthesis what is the drill?

1. Inspection.
2. Palpation.
3. Move.
4. X-ray.

With spondylolisthesis, what is seen on inspection? Give three features.

1. The transverse loin creases stand out.
2. The sacrum seems to extend to the waist.
3. The lumbar spine is short and on a plane in front of the sacrum.

What would one expect to feel with spondylolisthesis?

A step in the spinous processes posteriorly.

What about movement with spondylolisthesis?

They are either normal or all restricted.

In what way is the conservative management of spondylolisthesis related to conservative management of prolapsed lumbar intervertebral disc?

They are much the same.

Give three ways of fusing a spine in spondylolisthesis.

1. Interbody fusion.
2. Intertransverse fusion.
3. Posterior fusion.

Tumours Causing Backache

Classify tumours of this area into three groups.

1. Tumours of the spinal cord.
2. Tumours involving nerve root.
3. Tumours of the spinal column.

Tumours of the spinal cord are rare, and usually known as ..... .

Gliomas.

Since the cord is surrounded by meninges, one would also expect a ..... .

Meningioma.

Another tumour involving the cord or nerve root would be the ..... .

Neurofibroma.

Benign tumours of the vertebral column would include three:
namely ....., ... and
....

Chondroma, osteoclastoma
Vertebral haemangioma.

Primary malignant tumours include multiple myeloma and primary sarcoma.

Name five common secondary tumours.

Tumours arising from:
1. Thyroid.
2. Breast.
3. Prostate.
4. Kidney.
5. Lung.

Clinical features of the tumours are divided into three groups. What are they?

1. Compression of spinal cord.
2. Local destruction of the skeleton.
3. Interference with peripheral nerve.

Compression of the spinal cord eventually gives rise to a paralysis known as ..... with complete ..... and ..... loss, below the line of lesion.

Paraplegia.
Motor; Sensory.

Below the level of this lesion, we have an upper motor neurone lesion that has five main features when the lower limbs are examined. What are they?

1. Up-going toes, i.e. positive Babinski sign.
2. Lead-pipe rigidity.
3. Increased reflexes.
4. Clonus — ankle or knee.
5. Bladder and bowel dysfunction.

With the lower motor neurone lesion, what part of the spinal cord is involved?

The anterior horn cells.

Where there is local destruction of the spine, we might feel ..... and ..... .

Deformity; Swelling.

Where there is interference with a peripheral nerve, we would expect to get malfunction of the motor sensory and reflex phenomena related to the nerve root.

How many X-rays help in the diagnosis of back pain due to a tumour? Give six ways.

1. The radiograph of the spine might show a lesion within a vertebral body.
2. The radiograph of the spine might show a tumour eroding the bone from without.
3. The myelogram will show tumours of the cord.
4. Radiographs of the chest may reveal a primary lung tumour.
5. Radiographs of the rest of the skeleton may be helpful in excluding myeloma.
6. An I.V.P. may exclude a renal tumour.

The most modern way of diagnosing a bone tumour, of course, is with a bone ..... .

Scan.

Name three blood investigations that would help in diagnosing tumours that could cause low back pain.

1. E.S.R. is usually elevated with any type of tumour.
2. White cell count is elevated with leukaemia.
3. Serum acid phosphatase is elevated with prostatic tumours.

Which urine test can help with tumour investigation?

Bence Jones proteins are usually present in the urine of patients with myelomatosis.

With tumours of the spinal cord, what C.S.F. changes are noted?

C.S.F. protein is elevated.

Vascular Disorders Simulating Sciatica

* Peripheral vascular disease may sometimes simulate sciatica. In intermittent claudication, where may the obstruction lie?

1. In the iliac artery.
2. In the femoral artery.
3. In the popliteal artery.

* With claudication what induces the pain in the legs?

Exercise.

* What relieves it?

Cessation of exercise, namely resting the limb.

* What four pulses would you feel in order to exclude claudication?

1. Dorsalis pedis.
2. Posterior tibial artery.
3. Popliteal artery.
4. Femoral artery.

* With peripheral vascular disease, what happens to the skin temperature?

The skin is cold.

* If there be any doubts about the patient having sciatica or intermittent claudication, name three investigations to elucidate the problem.

1. Plain radiograph of the leg might show calcified popliteal artery.
2. Doppler examination of peripheral circulation.
3. Arteriography of the lower limb will reveal a blockage.

Sciatica and Back Pain Can Sometimes be Confused with Osteoarthritis of a Hip Joint

* How would you locate the pain of the arthritic hip?

The pain runs from groin anteriorly down the thigh to the front of the knee.

* What aggravates it?

Walking up or down steps or a slope.

* Hip joint movements are restricted in osteoarthritis. Name six hip joint movements.

1. Flexion.
2. Extension.
3. Abduction.
4. Adduction.
5. Internal rotation.
6. External rotation.

* Gynaecological causes of backache can be excluded by two examinations. What are they?

1. P.V.
2. P.R.

Ankylosing Spondylitis — See Chapter 29

CHAPTER 38

CAPSULITIS OR FROZEN SHOULDER

* Give two other names for frozen shoulder.

1. Adhesive capsulitis.
2. Peri arthritis.

* Is frozen shoulder common or rare?

It is very common.

* Which joint is involved?

Gleno-humeral joint.

* What are the two outstanding features of capsulitis or frozen shoulder?

1. Pain in the shoulder joint.
2. Limitation of movements.

* Whence does the pain radiate?

To deltoid insertion.

* What is the usual course of this disease?

A very slow spontaneous recovery that might take up to eighteen months.

Cause of Frozen Shoulder

* What is the cause?

It is unknown. Perhaps an autoimmune response to local tissue breakdown.

* Does injury play a part?

Not always.

* Does infection play a part?

No.

Pathology

* What part of the joint is involved?

The capsule.

* What happens to the capsule?

There is a loss of resilience.

* Is the mechanics of this understood?

No.

* Is the rigidity in the capsule reversible?

Yes. In almost every case eventually the condition returns to normal, i.e. the shoulder joint movements return to a full range.

What microscopic changes are seen in the capsule?

It is infiltrated with plasma cells and lymphocytes.

Clinical Features

* Of what does the patient complain?

Increasing pain and stiffness in shoulder joint.

What is the common age group?

Over 40 years.

* Physical examination reveals restriction of all gleno-humeral ..... .

Movements.

* Name the movements of the shoulder joint.

Abduction.
Flexion, extension and rotation (internal and external).

To what extent are the shoulder joint movements restricted?

To about a quarter or half the normal range.

In a severe case, most of the shoulder movements that remain are contributed by ..... movements.

Scapular.

* What do the radiographs show?

No abnormality.

* How long does a frozen shoulder take to recover?

Six-twelve months.

From what does one have to distinguish this condition?

Osteoarthritis or rheumatoid arthritis, both of which conditions are very rare in the shoulder.

* What are the main distinguishing features of a frozen shoulder?

Pain in the shoulder plus limitation of all glenohumeral movements without evidence of inflammation or destructive changes.

Treatment

* What is the best form of treatment of frozen shoulder in its early stages?

Sling immobilization with gentle exercises for short periods each day and reassure the patient that recovery is certain.

* How else may the pain be controlled?

By analgesic drugs and anti-inflammatory drugs.

* As the pain lessens, the exercises should be ..... .

Intensified.

* What type of heat might be used to help improve range of movement?

Shortwave diathermy.

Do ice packs help?

Yes, sometimes as effective as heat.

* Is manipulation ever indicated?

Yes, if the return of motion is slow it might be accelerated in this way after the acute pain has subsided.

* Manipulation may give rise to extreme ..... after the procedure has been completed.

Pain.

* How is this pain relieved?

By injecting local anaesthetic into the joint at the time of manipulation which, incidentally, is performed under a general anaesthetic.

What should follow the manipulation?

Exercises must be continued preferably under the supervision of a physiotherapist.

Name another intra-articular injection that may help.

Hydrocortisone acetate mixed with local anaesthetic.

CHAPTER 39

OLECRANON BURSITIS AND EPICONDYLITIS

* What is the name of the bursa behind the olecranon?

The olecranon bursa.

* Give three types of inflammation that might involve the olecranon bursa?

1. Traumatic bursitis.
2. Septic bursitis.
3. Gout.

* What is the other name of traumatic bursitis?

Student's elbow.

* In student's elbow with what is the bursa distended?

Clear fluid.

* Give one method of treating traumatic bursitis.

By aspiration followed by injection of hydrocortisone into the bursa.

* Should swelling persist, what treatment would you recommend for traumatic bursitis?

Excision of bursa.

Septic Bursitis

* Septic bursitis — how is that treated?

By adequate drainage followed by excision of bursa, and administration of appropriate antibiotics.

* Gouty bursitis is featured by having what type of crystals in the bursa?

Sodium biurate (tophi).

* Epicondylitis

Define epicondylitis.

A common painful affliction of the elbow associated with localised epicondylar tenderness on either medial or lateral sides.

What is the other name for epicondylitis?

Tennis elbow.

Where is the pain and tenderness located in this condition?

At the origin of the extensor or flexor muscles of the forearm.

What is the cause of tennis elbow?

Excessive use of the extensor muscles.

Is it always related to tennis?

No. Other activities are more frequently responsible.

What is thought to be the pathology of tennis elbow?

Incomplete rupture of aponeurotic fibres at the muscle origin.

Is this region plentifully supplied with nerve endings or not?

Plentifully supplied with nerve endings.

Can the elbow joint itself be affected with tennis elbow?

Yes. A rare cause of this condition can be a fringe of synovial membrane being caught up in the proximal radio-ulnar joint.

Where is the pain located in tennis elbow?

Lateral aspect of the elbow, i.e. at lateral epicondyle is the commonest site.

Is the medial epicondyle ever involved?

Yes.

Whence does the pain radiate?

Down the forearm.

Where else may the tenderness be located?

In the front of the lateral epicondyle of the humerus.

What makes the pain worse? Give three.

1. Putting the extensor muscles on the stretch, e.g. palmar flexing the wrist and fingers with the forearm pronated and the elbow extended.
2. Shaking hands.
3. Turning door knob.

* What do the radiographs show?

No abnormality.

* Resisted dorsi flexion gives rise to .... .

Pain.

* Left alone the condition usually ..... .

Subsides.

* For how long might the condition last?

One or two years.

Treatment

* What might be injected into the tender area?

Hydrocortisone.

* Sometimes it is preferable to inject the tender area first with .... before giving hydrocortisone injections.

Local anaesthetic.

* Whereabouts does one inject the local anaesthetic and hydrocortisone?

Directly into the most tender area.

* If hydrocortisone and local anaesthetic fails, give three physiotherapeutic methods that might succeed.

1. Shortwave diathermy.
2. Deep massage.
3. Faradic stimulation to extensor muscles.

* Does manipulation play a part in treatment?

Yes. This stretches the extensor muscles and may be used with or without local anaesthetic.

* When all else fails give another form of treatment.

Plaster of paris immobilization including elbow and wrist for six weeks.

* What is the essence of operative treatment?

In very resistant cases the extensor origin might be detached from the epicondyle with an osteotome.

CHAPTER 40

FRICTIONAL NEURITIS OF THE ULNA NERVE

The ulnar nerve is vulnerable behind the medial epicondyle of the humerus. Give two factors that can irritate the ulnar nerve in that position.

1. Osteoarthritis with encroachment of osteophytes.
2. Cubitus valgus: increased carrying angle, secondary to supracondylar fracture of the humerus in childhood.

What is the other name for the latter type of ulnar neuritis caused by a delayed effect of supracondylar fracture?

Tardy ulnar palsy.

In both these cases of friction neuritis, what change takes place in the ulnar nerve?

It undergoes fibrosis.

Can this fibrotic change become permanent?

Yes, if it is not relieved at an early stage.

Clinical Features of Frictional Neuritis of Ulnar Nerve

Where would you expect the numbness to be?

There is numbness along the ulnar border of the hand and the little finger and the medial half of the ring finger.

What motor changes would you expect in this condition in the hand?

Wasting and weakness of ulnar innervated small hand muscles.

Name these muscles.

The weakness would be in the muscles of the hypothenar eminence and all the interossei and the medial two lumbricals and the adductor of the thumb.

Name the two muscles the ulnar nerve supplies in the front of the forearm.

1. Flexor carpi ulnaris.
2. The medial half of flexor digitorum profundus.

Would these two muscles be weakened?

Yes.

What about skin sweating?

The skin in ulnar territory is drier than normal.

How may electromyographic studies help in diagnosis?

The ulnar innervated muscles may show partial denervation before motor signs are evident clinically.

What is the best method of treatment?

Transplant the ulnar nerve to the front of the joint.

CHAPTER 41

CARPAL TUNNEL SYNDROME

* Define carpal tunnel syndrome.

Carpal tunnel syndrome is a condition in which the median nerve, where it lies in front of the wrist, is compressed, giving rise to pins and needles in the nerve's sensory distribution and weakness of those muscles it supplies.

* Name the ligament that compresses the median nerve in front of the wrist.

The flexor retinaculum or anterior carpal ligament.

* Is the condition commoner in men or women?

Women — six times more common than in men.

* Is it commoner in young people or middle-aged people?

Middle-aged people.

* Give possible causes of carpal tunnel syndrome.

1. Thickening of tendon sheaths.
2. Osteoarthritis of the wrist.
3. Thickening of anterior carpal ligament following fracture of lower end of radius.
4. Myxoedema — general swelling of tissues.
5. Fluid retention, e.g. during pregnancy.

* In many cases, the cause of carpal tunnel syndrome remains ..... .

Undiscovered.

* If the retinaculum in ..... of the wrist is incised, the nerve can move ..... .

Front.
Forward.

* Why is the ulnar nerve not involved?

Because it does not pass behind the flexor retinaculum.

Clinical Features

* Since the median nerve has motor and sensory elements, one would expect both these parts of the nerve to be involved in the carpal tunnel syndrome.

* What are the sensory elements?

Tingling, numbness or discomfort in certain fingers.

* Which fingers?

Radial two and a half fingers and the thumb.

* What motor malfunction might be observed or complained of?

Clumsiness in carrying out fine movements, e.g. sewing.

* Is the tingling worse at night or day time?

Night time. Patient is frequently awakened in the early hours by pins and needles and pain.

* On examining a patient with carpal tunnel syndrome, what would one expect to find in the sensory field?

Blunting of sensation in median distribution.

* Later on, the sensory loss becomes more apparent and the motor wasting and weakness is also seen in median-innervated small muscles.

* What are the median-innervated small muscles of the hand?

Muscles of the thenar eminence and the outer two lumbricals (lateral or radial).

* Do you know any tests that may help in the diagnosis?

Yes, electrical tests may show decreased conduction velocity in the affected part of the median nerve.

Name this test.

The E.M.G. i.e. Electromyogram.

How may symptoms be reproduced?

By applying a sphygmomanometer cuff or by tapping over the carpal tunnel.

* The condition of carpal tunnel syndrome must be distinguished from three other conditions. What are they?

1. Cervical disc prolapse.
2. Brachial plexus lesions.
3. Cervical spondylosis.

Treatment

* What is the treatment of carpal tunnel syndrome?

Dividing the flexor retinaculum, thereby decompressing the nerve.

Name two less successful conservative methods.

1. Cock-up splint.
2. Injecting hydrocortisone into the flexor sheath.

CHAPTER 42

* DE QUERVAIN'S TENOVAGINITIS, TRIGGER FINGER AND GANGLION

* Define De Quervain's tenovaginitis.

De Quervain's tenovaginitis is a painful non-infective inflammation of certain wrist tendons causing pain on thumb movements.

* Give another name for De Quervain's teno-vaginitis.

Tenovaginitis of the abductor pollicis longus and extensor pollicis brevis tendons.

* Over what part of the radius is the tenderness?

Over styloid process.

* Thickening can be palpated over which two tendons?

Abductor pollicis longus and extensor pollicis brevis tendons.

What is the cause of De Quervain's tenovaginitis?

Unknown. Perhaps excessive friction from over-use as when wringing clothes.

* What is the pathology of the condition?

Thickening of fibrous sheaths of the two said tendons at the tip of the radial styloid process.

* Are the tendons themselves normal?

Yes.

Clinical Features

* The condition is commonest in which sex?

Female.

* The pain of De Quervain's is worsened by moving which tendons?

Abductor pollicis longus and extensor pollicis brevis.

* Give an example of these two tendons being activated.

Lifting a teapot.

Physical Examination

* Where is tenderness maximum in this condition?

At the radial styloid process.

* Can the thickened fibrous sheath be palpated?

Yes.

* Is passive adduction of the wrist or thumb conducive to increasing the pain?

Yes.

What clinical test is used in the diagnosis of De Quervain's tenovaginitis?

Findlestein's test: with the thumb enclosed within the flexed fingers the wrist is passively deviated in an ulnar direction. A positive result is indicated when sharp pain is felt over the radial styloid.

* Give three methods of treatment for De Quervain's tenovaginitis.

1. Do nothing and let nature cure it.
2. Inject hydrocortisone.
3. Incise the offending tendon sheath.

* Which of the three gives the best result?

Surgery, i.e. tendon sheath incision.

Trigger Finger

* Define trigger finger.

Trigger finger is a flexor tendon malfunction that prevents extension of the already flexed finger.

* Give two other names for trigger finger.

1. Digital tenovaginitis stenosans.
2. Snapping finger.

* Whereabouts is the constriction which causes difficulty with the extension of the flexed finger?

The fibrous digital sheath interferes with the free flow of the contained flexor tendon. The actual obstruction takes place in the palm of the hand adjacent to or in front of the meta-carpal neck.

* If a fibrous sheath is constricted, what happens to the contained tendon?

It becomes swollen.

* What is the main difficulty with trigger finger?

The fully flexed finger has a problem trying to be extended because the swollen part of the tendon becomes caught in the constricted part of the fibrous sheath.

* The condition occurs in two types of persons. What are they?

In the fingers of middle aged people, usually women, and in infants.

The Adult Type

* Where is the tenderness located in the adult?

At the base of the affected finger.

* What is the other complaint?

Locking of the finger in full flexion.

How is the locking overcome? Give two methods.

By supreme effort to extend the finger on the patient's part, or by extending the finger passively with the other hand.

Physical Examination

* Palpation at finger base or in the palm reveals a ....

Nodule.

* This nodule is ..... .

Tender.

* The tenderness is at the ..... of the fibrous sheath.

Mouth.

* Is it possible to reproduce the snapping with passive movement?

No, only when the patient flexes the finger fully with his own muscle does the snapping take place.

The Infantile Type

Which digit is the commonest?

The thumb.

The infant is unable to straighten the thumb which is locked in ..... .

Flexion.

Whereabouts does one feel the nodule in the thumb of infants in this condition?

At the base of the thumb in the position of the mouth of the fibrous flexor sheath.

Give another landmark for this nodule.

At the head of the metacarpal bone.

Give two conditions that could simulate trigger thumb defect in children.

1. A dislocated thumb.
2. Congenital deformity.

Treatment

In early cases what treatment may be effective?

The injection of hydrocortisone into the entrance of the tendon sheath.

What is the best form of treatment in both adult and infantile types?

Incision of fibrous flexor sheath at the thickened part.

Why would you delay surgery in the infantile type?

Because spontaneous recovery may occur.

Ganglion

Whence do ganglia arise?

From small bursae within the substance of the joint capsule or the fibrous tendon sheath.

What age is the patient?

Usually a young adult presents with a painless lump.

What is the commonest site of a ganglion?

The back of the wrist.

What is the best form of treatment for a ganglion?

The ganglion should be removed surgically, or by aspiration with a large bored needle.

CHAPTER 43

DUPUYTREN'S CONTRACTURE

* Define Dupuytren's contracture.

This is a condition in which fibrotic contracture of the palmar fascia produces flexion deformity of certain fingers causing the digits to be contracted into the palm of the hand.

* What is the other name for this condition?

Contracture of palmar aponeurosis.

* Thickening and shortening of the ..... aponeurosis gives rise to a ..... contracture of one or more of the fingers.

Palmar.
Flexion.

* With regard to cause of Dupuytren's contracture, does heredity play a part?

Yes.

* The significance of injury is ..... .

Uncertain.

* There is an increased incidence of the disorder amongst ..... .

Epileptics.

Name two other diseases in which it is commonly seen.

1. Alcoholic cirrhosis.
2. Diabetes.

Pathology

* Give the other name for the palmar aponeurosis.

Palmar fascia.

* Where is the proximal attachment of this fascia?

It merges with the palmaris longus tendon at the front of the wrist.

* Where is the distal attachment of this fascia?

Into the proximal and middle phalanges of the fingers.

* Of all the layers of the palm of the hand, the palmar fascia lies immediately behind which one?

The skin.

* In Dupuytren's contracture, two changes take place in the aponeurosis. What are they?

1. The aponeurosis becomes greatly thickened, perhaps more than half a centimetre.
2. The aponeurosis contracts, thus pulling the involved fingers into the palm of the hand.

* Considering the distal attachment of the palmar aponeurosis, which joints would be flexed with the contracting process?

1. The metacarpo-phalangeal joint.
2. The proximal inter-phalangeal joint.

* Which half of the aponeurosis is more commonly affected?

The ulnar half.

* Therefore, which are the commoner fingers to be involved?

The little and ring fingers.

* With long established Dupuytren's contracture, what happens to the capsule of the two said joints?

The capsule undergoes contracture on the volar aspect thus preventing extension of finger or fingers either actively or passively.

* Does the condition ever appear in the feet?

Yes.

* In what way does the foot Dupuytren's differ from the hand Dupuytren's?

Actual contracture of the toes is very rare in the foot Dupuytren's.

Clinical Features of Dupuytren's Contracture

* Is this condition more common in men or women?

Men.

* Is it usual for one or two hands to be involved?

Two.

Describe the palm.

Puckered and nodular with obvious subcutaneous cords.

* Where is the first sign of Dupuytren's usually noticed?

In the mid-palm, opposite the base of the ring finger.

* Does the skin ever get attached to the fascial bands?

Yes.

Treatment of Dupuytren's Contracture

* There are three lines of approach in the treatment of Dupuytren's contracture. What are they?

1. In very elderly people, do nothing.
2. Careful wide excision of the palmar aponeurosis.
3. Simple division of the taut contracted band is usually unsatisfactory.

In the elderly, a finger of nuisance stuck in the palm may require ..... .

Amputation.

* What is the main complication of the operation (No. 2 above)?

Damage to the cutaneous nerves.

How do you manage the hand after these operations?

Splint fingers straight between physiotherapy sessions that last for six weeks.

CHAPTER 44

CONGENITAL DISLOCATION OF THE HIP

* Define congenital dislocation of the hip.

A condition in which a baby is born with one or both femoral heads displaced out of the acetabulum.

* This is a spontaneous dislocation: does it occur before, during or after birth?

It can occur either before, during or shortly after birth.

* Give two reasons for its great importance.

1. It is the commonest of congenital deformities.
2. If it is missed or undiagnosed or neglected or inefficiently treated, it leaves the patient with a life-long crippling deformity.

Causes

An important factor is joint laxity. Give two explanations for this.

1. General ligamentous laxity is found and may be present in the parents.
2. Hormonal joint laxity. In females, a ligament relaxing hormone may be secreted by the foetal uterus in response to hormones reaching the foetal circulation from the mother.

* Why is the condition commoner in girls than boys?

Because the foetal uterus produces relaxin — this is just a theory.

May C.D.H. be related to breech delivery?

Yes, there is a slightly greater incidence of dislocation with breech delivery.

Pathology

* Name three features seen on an antero-posterior radiograph in C.D.H.

1. The retarded development of the capital epiphysis.
2. Steeply sloping acetabulum roof.
3. Lateral and upward displacement of the upper end of the femur.

What happens to the femoral neck?

It is anteverted, i.e. the neck is directed too far forward.

What might happen to the labrum or limbus of the acetabulum?

It might be folded into the cavity of the acetabulum.

What happens to the capsule as the femoral head is displaced upwards?

It becomes elongated.

What happens to the labrum or limbus in C.D.H.?

It is folded into the cavity of the acetabulum thus preventing the head from being seated in the acetabulum.

What problem does the limbus create?

It makes reduction of the dislocation difficult.

Clinical Features

* Is it commoner in boys or girls?

Five times commoner in girls.

* In what percentage of cases are both hips affected?

Thirty-three percent.

If the condition is not specifically sought shortly after birth, what might happen?

The abnormality may not be noticed until the child begins to walk.

* Give two features that might be noticed in a case of missed C.D.H. when the child walks.

1. Walking is delayed.
2. There is a limp or waddling gait.

* On looking at the buttocks of a baby with C.D.H., what do we see?

Asymmetry of the buttock folds and shortening of the affected limb.

* In bilateral cases, what do we notice about the perineum?

It is widened.

What about the curves in the spine?

In C.D.H., there is an exaggeration, i.e. there is a deep hollow in the back. Joint movements are full except for abduction.

What is meant by the telescopic movement?

Abnormal mobility in long axis of femur.

Radiographic Examination

* Give three main radiographic features.

1. Ossific centre of head of femur late in appearing.
2. Bony acetabular roof slopes upward.
3. The femoral head as judged by ossific centre is displaced upwards and laterally.

Name a special radiograph that will show the defect inside the joint.

Arthrography.

What is Ortolani's sign?

With the hip and knees flexed to ninety degrees and the baby lying supine, the process of abducting the hip joint produces a click as the dislocated hip slips into the acetabulum, thus reducing.

Give an important clinical sign in children 1—2 years of age with C.D.H.

There is restriction of range of abduction when the hip is flexed.

If there be any doubt in a two year old who is slow to walk or walks with an abnormal gait, what would you recommend?

Insist on radiographic examination.

Name two important factors in prognosis.

Early detection and reduction.

Of patients who are missed in the first year of life, what percentage ultimately get a trouble-free hip joint?

Between fifty and sixty-six percent of these people would be trouble free, after appropriate treatment.

* What is the complication that occurs in middle adult life in undiagnosed cases?

Osteoarthritis.

What is the prognosis in children who are diagnosed and treated within the first week of life?

Excellent result to be expected.

Treatment — Neo-Natal Cases

Neo-natal cases range from birth to how many months?

Six months of age.

How is the dislocation reduced in these early cases?

By simply abducting the hip.

How is the abduction maintained?

By a splint or by plaster of paris that holds the hip or hips flexed and abducted to ninety degrees.

For how long are the hips held in abduction?

Three months.

How do we check that the head is still in the acetabulum?

By periodical radiographic checks up to the age of a year.

Treatment — Six Months to Three Years

Non-operative treatment: this is less common or more common than before?

Non-operative treatment is less common, i.e. more surgeons operate.

The non-operative treatment: how is the dislocation reduced?

By weight traction followed by gentle manipulation.

What is the purpose of traction?

Gradually to stretch the soft tissues to bring the femoral head down to the level of the acetabulum.

What must you do to reduce the head when it is level with the acetabulum?

Gradually abduct a little each day till ninety degrees of abduction is reached.

In young children, this can be successful. If reduction has not occurred after traction for four weeks, what will you do?

Do a gentle manipulation under anaesthesia and this will probably succeed.

How do you hold the head reduced in the acetabulum?

With a plaster of paris hip spica with the hip joints in eighty degrees of abduction.

Is it wise or unwise to have the hips medially rotated as well?

Wise. Medial rotation is quite good although some surgeons prefer lateral rotation.

For how long is splintage continued?

For nine months to a year.

What happens to the acetabulum during this process?

It increases in depth.

What treatment is necessary after that?

No treatment.

Operative Treatment — Six Months to Three Years

If the head won't stay in the acetabulum what is the most likely reason?

The acetabulum may be filled with the limbus thus preventing reduction.

What is the other name for the limbus?

The acetabular labrum.

Give an indication then for surgery in this age group.

The limbus obstructing reduction requires surgical excision.

The problem of excessive anteversion. How is this treated?

By rotational osteotomy below the greater trochanter.

In which direction is the femoral shaft rotated?

Laterally, in relation to the upper end of the femur.

When would this operation be advised?

About a month after the dislocation has been reduced.

What is the purpose of this operation?

To correct excessive anteversion of the femoral neck.

In the age group, six months to three years, what would you do if recurrence of dislocation or subluxation took place?

An operation would be necessary to improve the shape and depth of the acetabulum or the disposition of the acetabulum would have to be altered.

Name three such operations that would achieve these points.

1. Acetabuloplasty.
2. Salter's operation (innominate osteotomy).
3. Chiari's pelvic osteotomy.

What is an acetabuloplasty?

In this operation, a rim of bone and cartilage is levered out of the ilium to widen the acetabular roof and make it more horizontal.

What is done with the resulting gap left above the acetabulum?

This wedge shaped space is filled wirh a bone graft.

What is the other name for this operation?

The shelf operation.

What is the other name for Salter's operation?

Osteotomy of the innominate bone.

What is the extent of the osteotomy in this operation?

From immediately above the acetabulum to the greater sciatic notch.

As the whole of the lower half of the bone is sprung downwards, on what is it hinged?

On the symphysis pubis.

What effect does Salter's operation have on the acetabulum?

It redirects it so it is pointing more directly downwards. In this way, the hip joint is made more stable.

In Chiari's pelvic displacement osteotomy, where is the iliac bone divided?

Immediately above the acetabulum.

In which direction is it divided?

Transversely.

The lower fragment bearing the acetabulum is displaced in which direction?

Medially.

The extension of the acetabular roof comprises what structure?

The cut surface of the upper fragment forms an extension to the acetabular roof with capsule and newly formed fibrous tissue intervening.

Is the tendency nowadays to operate more or less than previously?

More surgeons are tending to operate now than they did previously.

In this age group, what are the advantages of surgery?

The ensuring of perfect reduction of the dislocation can be obtained by the Salter operation combined with the rotational osteotomy to correct the anteversion. The results seem so good that most people think that it is worthwhile proceeding directly to it in this age group.

Congenital Dislocation of the Hip — Four to Eight Years

Is conservative treatment likely to be successful after the age of three?

No.

If reduction is to be attempted, how should it be done?

By open reduction.

In these late cases, what is the acetabulum like?

Usually poorly developed.

What does this mean?

It usually means that a reconstructive operation like those described above has to be undertaken.

If excessive anteversion of the femoral neck is present, what would be required?

Rotation osteotomy.

Is this usually necessary?

Yes.

Age Nine Years Onwards

After the age of nine years what are the indications for surgery?

A painful secondary degenerative change in the hip joint.

If one hip is affected with painful degeneration, what operation would you recommend?

Arthrodesis.

If both hips are affected with painful degeneration after the age of nine, what operation can be done?

Abduction osteotomy of the femur at the level of the ischial tuberosity.

What is the name of this operation?

Schanz.

How does this operation work?

It eliminates the Trendelenburg dip on walking.

The stability of the hip is further improved by the .... of the femoral shaft.

Medial shift.

CHAPTER 45

PERTHES' DISEASE

* Define Perthes' disease.

An affection of obscure origin involving the head of the femur of children in the 5—10 age group and causing groin pain and a limp.

Give four other names for Perthes' disease.

1. Legg-Perthes' disease.
2. Coxa-plana disease.
3. Pseudo-coxalgia.
4. Osteochondritis of the femoral capital epiphysis.

* In what age group do we find Perthes' disease?

Five-ten years.

* In the early stages, what happens to the femoral head?

It becomes softened and perhaps deformed.

What is the main problem in the long-term that we have to think of with Perthes' disease?

It may proceed to osteoarthritis of the hip in later life.

What is the cause of Perthes' disease?

Unknown.

* What part does blood supply play?

A local disturbance of blood supply is believed to play a part in Perthes' disease.

Pathology

What happens to the bony nucleus?

The bony nucleus of the epiphysis undergoes necrosis and loses its trabecular structure.

It becomes softened, i.e. the nucleus of the epiphysis becomes softened and weight bearing, therefore, has what effect?

The bony nucleus then becomes flattened with weight bearing.

After this phase, what happens to the bone?

It becomes re-vascularized and hardened.

Apley says that between four and seven the femoral head blood supply is derived mainly from .... and in the effused ..... these are cut off producing ....

Lateral epiphyseal vessels; Joint.
An avascular head.

The minor trauma causes an effusion which in turn blocks .... vessels.

Lateral epiphyseal.

The onset of symptoms is associated with minor trauma in .....% of cases.

50%.

* If the bony nucleus has been flattened, the hardening process leaves a permanently flat head thus giving rise to ..... .

Osteoarthritis (in the later stages).

How long do the phases of necrosis and re-vascularization take?

Two years or more.

As a result of Perthes' disease, what might happen to the femoral neck?

It may be permanently shorter than normal.

What happens normally to the femoral head after Perthes' disease?

It is usually enlarged.

Clinical Features

* Age group?

Five-ten years.

* Does it affect one hip more often than two hips?

Usually one hip.

* Of what does the child complain?

Pain in the groin.

* Is there a limp?

Yes.

Is general health impaired?

No.

Physical examination of the hip reveals three striking features on testing movements. What are they?

1. Limitation of all hip movements.
2. Pain with hip movements.
3. Spasm of the muscles.

The early radiographic examination shows a change in the ossific nucleus of the femoral head. What is it?

There is a slight decrease in depth of the ossific nucleus.

* What happens to the joint space?

It is increased in depth.

In other words, the bony nucleus seems to have ..... .

Shrunk.

There is an increase in ..... in the nucleus compared to the normal side.

Density.

What happens to the nucleus at a later stage?

It becomes fragmented in appearance.

If the head hardens up whilst in a flattened state, it ends up ..... and ..... .

Hard; Deformed.

What condition can simulate Perthes' disease?

Tuberculous arthritis.

Do the radiographs of Perthes' and tuberculous arthritis appear much the same?

Yes.

Give one way in which the two conditions can be distinguished.

The E.S.R. is raised in T.B. and not in Perthes' disease.

What is the single main complication that takes place with Perthes' disease in the fourth or fifth decade?

Osteoarthritis of the hip joint.

Is the prognosis more favourable in the younger child or in the older?

In the younger child it is more favourable.

Upon what single factor does the development of osteoarthritis in later life depend?

If the whole of the epiphysis is affected, osteoarthritis is more likely to occur than if only part of the epiphysis is involved.

Treatment of Perthes' Disease

In days gone by, what used to be the treatment?

Two years or more non-weight bearing with prolonged recumbency.

Why was this treatment abandoned?

Results were not commensurate with the severe disruption of home life.

* What is the principle of treatment?	To prevent pressure upon the head of the femur while still allowing the child to be up and about.
* Give two ways in which the head may be held completely contained in the acetabulum.	By abducting both hips and holding them in that position or by adduction osteotomy.

Abduction Apparatus

What is the purpose of this device?	To hold the hip abducted twenty-thirty degrees on each side. Some surgeons prefer surgery.

Osteotomy

At what point is the femur divided?	Below the greater trochanter.
In which direction is the shaft of the femur angled?	The shaft fragment is angled medially in relation to the proximal fragment.
When the leg is in the neutral position, the upper end of the femur (head and neck) is in what position?	Abducted. In this way, the long axis corresponds with the central axis of the acetabulum.
What is the angle of adduction at the osteotomy site?	About twenty degrees.
How are the fragments held?	With a metal nail plate and screws.
How long does union take to occur?	Five or six weeks.
When may walking be commenced?	After five or six weeks.

Prognosis in Perthes' Disease

* What significance do you attach to a lateral radiograph showing not more than half of the femoral head affected?	The prognosis here is good.
Would this mean that regardless of treatment, these patients do well?	Yes. An expectant policy may therefore be adopted in these cases.
If a larger part of the femoral head is affected, the outlook is	Poor.
In these cases, the femur is held in what position?	Abducted position.
What is the purpose of this?	To keep the whole of the epiphysis of the femoral head contained within the acetabulum.
Why is this thought to be beneficial?	So that the intact acetabulum will serve as a mould to preserve the shape of the femoral head during the process of re-vascularization.

CHAPTER 46

SLIPPED UPPER FEMORAL EPIPHYSIS AND
SALTER HARRIS EPIPHYSEAL PLATE INJURIES

* Define slipped upper femoral epiphysis.

A condition seen in the hip joints of adolescents in which the epiphysis of the upper end of the femur comes unstuck and slips off backwards.

Give two other names for this condition.

1. Adolescent coxavara.
2. Epiphyseal coxavara.

At what age does it manifest?

Late childhood, e.g. adolescence.

* What part of the upper femur is displaced?

The upper femoral epiphysis is displaced from its normal position upon the femoral neck.

* What is the cause of slipped upper femoral epiphysis?

Unknown. Thought to be an imbalance between the growth hormone and the sex hormone.

* Whereabouts is the loosening observed?

At the junction of the capital epiphysis and the neck of the femur.

* In which direction is the epiphysis displaced?

Downwards and backwards.

* What makes the epiphysis pass downwards?

Weight bearing.

What makes the epiphysis go backwards?

The forward pull of the muscles attached to the upper femur, e.g. ilio psoas.

Does the backward displacement of the femoral epiphysis take place gradually or suddenly?

It may be either suddenly as in a fall, or gradually.

In what % is it gradual?

70%.

Therefore in what % is it sudden?

30%.

What would happen if the displaced epiphysis is not reduced correctly?

The epiphysis would fuse to the femoral neck in the abnormal position.

A permanently displaced epiphysis in later years may give rise to ..... .

Osteoarthritis (but **not** always).

Clinical Features

Is it commoner in boys or girls?

Boys — slightly more common.

* What is the usual age range?

Ten-fifteen years.

Give two common symptoms.

1. Groin pain following minor injury.
2. Limp.

What percentage of these boys have the "fat boy or Dickens" type of build?

Fifty percent.

In what percentage of cases are both hips affected?

Fifty percent.

May both hips be affected simultaneously or consecutively?

Consecutively.

* Is it usual to have gradual onset of pain in the hip or sudden onset?

Gradual onset is the usual thing.

* Is the pain sometimes referred to the knee?

Yes.

Is it common or rare for symptoms to develop acutely after an injury?

Rare.

Physical Examination

Certain hip movements are restricted. Name three.

Flexion, abduction and medial rotation are all restricted.

Name two movements that are increased in range.

Lateral rotation and adduction.

* In which direction does the limb tend to lie when the patient is supine and relaxed.

In lateral rotation.

What about limb length?

With a significant slip there may be 1–2 cm of shortening.

Radiographic Examination

* Which radiograph gives the better diagnostic picture, the lateral or the antero-posterior?

The lateral.

* A slight displacement is easily ..... if a-p films alone are examined.

Overlooked.

What is Trethowan's sign?

In a-p view a line drawn along the superior surface of the neck remains superior to the head instead of passing through it.

* In the lateral film, what happens to the epiphysis?

It is tilted over toward the back of the femoral neck, the posterior horn being lower than the anterior horn.

Diagnosis

* Slipped epiphysis should be suspected in every patient between ..... and ..... who complains of pain in the ..... or ..... .

Ten; Fifteen.
Hip; Knee.

* The all important radiographic evidence is that of the slip seen on the ..... radiograph.

Lateral.

Treatment

* How do you define a slight slip?

One in which there is less than 1 cm of slip as seen on the radiographs.

* Slight slip is treated in what fashion?

All that is necessary is to prevent further displacement.

* How is this achieved?

By driving threaded wires or a screw along the neck of the femur into the epiphysis.

* When displacement is severe, why can it not be simply left?

Because of the high probability of osteoarthritis developing later in life.

When displacement is severe, there are three modes of attack. What are they?

1. Manipulation and internal fixation.
2. Operative replacement of the epiphysis.
3. Compensatory osteotomy at a lower level.

Manipulation: is this occasionally or frequently successful?

Occasionally.

Under what circumstances is it worth trying?

With a recent displacement or slip.

What is the risk of manipulation if it is not performed gently?

The blood supply to the epiphysis may be damaged.

After successful manipulation, how does one prevent further slip?

By the use of threaded wires or a screw.

At what point of time would you consider operative replacement of the epiphysis and internal fixation with wires or a screw?

When the condition has been present for less than three months?

Does this restore the hip to normal?

Yes, in most cases.

What is the disadvantage with this operation done in less than three monrhs.

Impairment of blood supply might lead to death of femoral head and osteoarthritis in later life.

Name an operation that can be performed particularly after the condition has been present for three months.

Compensatory osteotomy.

Where in the femur is the osteotomy carried out?

Just below the trochanteric level.

After three months, will the joint itself ever return to normal?

No, adaptive changes have occurred in the bone by then.

With the osteotomy operation, where is the wedge based?

It is an anteriorly based wedge of bone removed from the shaft of the femur.

Complications

* The outstanding complication in the long-term is ....

Avascular necrosis.

Give three factors that might produce damage to the blood supply, thus causing avascular necrosis.

1. Manipulation of the joint in an endeavour to replace the epiphysis.
2. Operation on the joint to replace the epiphysis.
3. Spontaneous avascular necrosis might take place.

* What is the main complication which takes place later in life if the displacement is allowed to remain?

Osteoarthritis usually develops in later life if the slip is uncorrected.

When one is concentrating on the hip on one side, we must beware of the ..... on the other side.

Hip — i.e. the opposite epiphysis may slip.

Compensatory Osteotomy

The anterior based wedge of bone is removed in order to achieve what?

To angle the shaft of the femur into flexion relative to the upper fragment.

Is it possible to rotate the shaft as well?

Yes.

In this way, the operation compensates for the backward ..... of the epiphysis.

Tilting.

What is the gauge which enables you to assess whether or not the compensation has been adequate?

Correction should be sufficient to bring the epiphysis once more into the weight transmitting segment of the acetabulum.

Does this operation of compensatory osteotomy endanger the blood supply of the femoral head?

No.

The articular surface of the upper end of the femur is still deformed, therefore, secondary ..... in later years is quite possible.

Osteoarthritis.

* There is general agreement that when the displacement is slight, it is best to accept the ..... .

Position.

* How might one prevent further slipping?

By inserting threaded wires across the epiphyseal line.

The Injuries Involving the Epiphyseal Plate

Whose names are associated with the classification of epiphyseal injuries?

Salter and Harris.

Each epiphysis has its own plate through which .... occurs.

Skeletal growth.

Name the two types of epiphyses that exist in the extremities.

1. Pressure epiphyses.
2. Traction epiphyses.

Where is the pressure epiphysis located?

At the ends of the long bones.

The epiphyseal plate adjacent to the epiphysis provides .... for the long bone.

Longitudinal growth.

The epiphyseal plate is situated between the ..... and ..... .

Epiphysis.
Metaphysis.

The traction epiphyses are subjected to ..... rather than to pressure.

Traction.

The traction epiphysis is located at the site of ..... or ..... of major muscles.

Origin; Insertion.

These traction epiphyses are therefore subjected to ..... rather than to ..... .

Traction; Pressure.

Does the traction epiphysis play any part in longitudinal growth of the bone?

No.

Does the pressure epiphysis play any part in longitudinal bone growth?

Yes.

Give two examples of traction epiphyses.

1. The lesser trochanter of the femur.
2. The medial epicondyle of the humerus.

The normal epiphyseal plate consists of four distinct layers. What are they?

1. The resting cells.
2. The proliferating cells.
3. The hypertrophying cells.
4. Endochondral ossification.

What fills the space between the cells?

Cartilage matrix or intercellular substance.

What part does the intercellular substance play in the epiphyseal plate?

It provides the strength.

The intercellular substance or cartilage matrix then rather than the cells provides the resistance to ..... .

Shear.

Whereabouts is the plane of cleavage after epiphyseal separation?

In the third layer, namely the hypertrophying cell layer where the matrix is scanty, thus making the plate weak.

With separation the growing cells remain attached to which part?

To the epiphysis.

If the blood supply to these cells is not damaged by the separation, normal ..... should continue satisfactorily.

Growth.

In the lower extremity whereabouts does longitudinal growth occur for the most part?

In the region of the knee.

In the upper extremity however, there is more longitudinal growth at the ..... and ..... than at the elbow.

Shoulder; Wrist.

Classification of Epiphyseal Plate Injuries

What is meant by a type one Salter Harris epiphyseal plate injury?

Here there is complete separation of the epiphysis from the metaphysis without any bone fracture.

With type one injuries, what happens to the growing cells of the epiphyseal plate?

The growing cells of the epiphyseal plate remain with the epiphysis.

Prognosis generally for future growth is ..... .

Excellent.

Give one example, however, where the blood supply to the epiphysis may be damaged thus causing retardation of growth.

At the upper end of the femur — here the epiphysis is entirely covered by cartilage and the blood supply is frequently damaged with consequent premature closure of the epiphyseal plate.

What is meant by a type two Salter Harris epiphyseal plate injury?

Here the line of separation extends along the epiphyseal plate for a variable distance and then out through a portion of the metaphysis — thus producing the familiar triangular shaped metaphyseal fragment.

Is this type two injury common or rare?

It is the commonest type of epiphyseal plate injury.

The growing cartilage cells of the epiphyseal plate remain where?

With the epiphysis. Thus the prognosis for growth is excellent.

What is a type three Salter Harris epiphyseal plate injury?

The fracture which is intra-articular extends from the joint surface to the weak zone of the epiphyseal plate and then extends along the plate to its periphery.

What is meant by a type four Salter Harris epiphyseal plate injury?

The fracture extends from the joint surface through the epiphysis across the full thickness of the epiphyseal plate and through a portion of the metaphysis thereby producing a complete split.

Give a common example of this type of injury.

Fracture of the lateral condyle of the humerus.

In these cases the epiphyseal plate must be accurately re-aligned in order to prevent bone union across the plate with resultant local premature cessation of growth, and this degree of accuracy is achieved with the aid of ....

Internal fixation.

What is meant by a type five epiphyseal plate injury?

This common injury results from a severe crushing force applied to one area of the epiphyseal plate.

Give an example of this type of injury.

A severe abduction injury to a joint such as the knee is likely to produce crushing of the epiphyseal plate.

Specific Epiphyseal Plate Injuries
Lower Radial Epiphysis

Epiphyseal injuries of the lower radius are almost invariably type ..... .

Two.

In reducing these injuries what prevents overcorrection?

The intact hinge of periosteum.

Whence should the plaster extend in these cases?

The plaster should extend above the elbow with the forearm pronated and the wrist in ulnar deviation and slightly palmar flexed.

For how long should the immobilisation be retained?

Three weeks.

Injuries of Upper Radial Epiphysis

What type are they usually?

Type two.

How is reduction achieved?

By direct pressure over the radial head through the closed skin.

Under what circumstances would you recommend opening the elbow to restore alignment of the upper radial epiphysis?

If there is more than 15 degrees residual angulation after closed reduction, open reduction should be undertaken.

Give two reasons why the radial head should never be excised in children.

1. The resultant loss of growth in the radius will produce progressive radial deviation at the wrist joint.
2. The resultant loss of growth in the radius inevitably produces progressive valgus deformity of the elbow.

Fracture of the lateral condyle of the humerus (capitulum) is usually a type ..... injury.

Four.

Is open reduction usually necessary?

Yes, if there is displacement.

Why is reduction of an accurate degree essential?

1. To restore a smooth joint.
2. To re-align the epiphyseal plate.

How may immobilisation be achieved?

Either by multiple sutures or by two fine removable Kirschner wires.

How would you immobilise the elbow after this procedure?

The elbow should be immobilised for three weeks at 90 degrees.

Premature cessation of growth due to impaired blood supply or inaccurate reduction would give rise to two serious complications, what are they?

1. Progressive valgus deformity of the elbow.
2. Tardy ulna nerve paralysis.

Upper Humeral Epiphyseal Injuries

Is perfect reduction essential?

No — because remodelling of the upper end of the humerus from the periosteal tube is very satisfactory.

Is open operation ever necessary?

No — very rarely.

Lower Tibial Epiphyseal Injuries

Are these injuries usually treated by closed or open reductions?

By closed reductions.

Are type three injuries at this level common or rare?

Common.

Is the type five injury common or rare in the lower tibial epiphyseal area?

It is very common.

Of all the epiphyses, which one is seen to exhibit an ossification centre at birth?

The lower femoral epiphysis.

With regard to knee injuries, which is the stronger, the epiphyseal plate or the ligaments?

The ligaments are stronger — therefore with the injury in the knee the slipping of the epiphysis is more commonly seen than ligamentous injuries.

What type are upper femoral epiphyseal injuries?

Type one.

Why is the prognosis poor?

Because the upper femoral epiphysis frequently loses its blood supply with a resultant avascular necrosis of the epiphysis.

Whence does the epiphyseal plate receive its nutrition?

From the epiphyseal side of the plate so that avascular necrosis of the femoral head results in death of epiphyseal plate and subsequent premature cessation of growth.

With regard to injuries involving traction epiphyses, it is essential to .... the adjacent muscle.

Replace.

Name four areas where one might see avulsion of the traction epiphysis.

1. Medial epicondyle of the humerus.
2. Tibial tubercle.
3. Lesser trochanter of the femur.
4. Traction epiphyses of the pelvis.

CHAPTER 47

* OSTEOARTHRITIS OF THE HIP

* Define osteoarthritis of the hip joint.

A painful condition of the hip seen usually in the elderly and associated with stiffness and deformity in that articulation.

* Is it commoner in elderly people or the younger age group?

Elderly people.

* What is the cause of osteoarthritis?

Wear and tear.

What two factors accelerate the wear and tear process?

1. Disease to the joint.
2. Injury to the joint.

* Give an example of two diseases of the joint that can cause osteoarthritis.

1. Perthes' disease.
2. Slipped upper femoral epiphysis.

* Give an example of injury to a joint causing osteoarthritis.

Fracture of the acetabulum.

* Give an example of a congenital abnormality that can cause osteoarthritis.

Congenital subluxation or dislocation of the hip.

Name two inflammatory conditions that may predispose to osteoarthritis.

1. Rheumatoid arthritis.
2. Septic arthritis.

Pathology

* What happens to the articular cartilage?

It is worn away.

What part of the articular cartilage is worn away?

The weight bearing part.

* The underlying bone becomes hard and ..... .

Eburnated.

What happens to the bone in the margin of the joint?

It undergoes hypertrophy.

In osteoarthritis, where is the pain situated?

In the groin.

* To what part does the pain radiate?

Front of thigh.

* Does it ever go as low as the knee?

Yes, often the patient thinks the problem is in the knee.

What is Protrusio Acetabuli?

A condition seen in women (more often) in which the acetabulum is sunken forming up to 2/3 of a sphere, the normal being 1/2.

What is its significance?

It is a precursor to osteoarthritis.

What makes the pain of an arthritic hip worse?

Walking.

What relieves the pain?

Rest.

As joint stiffness increases, give two manoeuvres the patient has difficulty performing.

1. Cutting toenails.
2. Tying shoelaces.

The symptoms increase month by month and the patient develops a severe ..... limp.

Painful.

Physical Examination

* What happens to hip joint movements?

All are restricted.

Which movements (name three) are the most affected?

Abduction, adduction and rotational movements.

Which movement might well be preserved?

Flexion is preserved for a considerable time.

* In what position is the hip joint in fixed deformity?

In flexion and adduction or lateral rotation or a combination of these.

* Give four radiographic manifestations of osteoarthritis of the hip joint.

1. Diminution of joint space.
2. Tendency towards sclerosis of the surface bone.
3. Hypertrophic spurring of bone (osteophyte formation).
4. Cyst formation.

Treatment

* Conservative treatment is discussed under four headings. What are they?

1. Relative rest.
2. Drugs.
3. Physiotherapy.
4. Injections into the joint (hydrocortisone).

* Give two examples of relative rest.

1. Alter way of life so that patient is sitting more than standing or walking.
2. Use of walking stick.

* Drugs — name four drugs that can be helpful.

1. Aspirin.
2. Indocid.
3. Naprosyn.
4. Butazolidine.

* Physiotherapy: give two forms of physiotherapy.

1. Shortwave diathermy.
2. Exercises to strengthen the muscles and to preserve mobility.

Injections into the joint: what could be injected?

Hydrocortisone plus local anaesthetic.

Operative Treatment

What is the main indication?

Increasing pain and deformity at the hip joint.

* Name four types of operation used for osteoarthritis of the hip joint.

1. Arthroplasty: replacement arthroplasty and excision arthroplasty.
2. McMurray osteotomy.
3. Arthrodesis.
4. Muscle release — rare.

Replacement Arthroplasty

* With this operation, what happens to the femoral head?

It is excised and replaced by a metal prosthesis.

* How is the prosthesis held in position?

By acrylic cement.

* What is done about the acetabulum in total hip replacement or replacement arthroplasty?

It is fitted with a high density polyethylene cup.

* How is this plastic cup held rigidly in the acetabulum?

By acrylic cement.

* The insertion of these two components constitutes a phenomenon known as ....

Total replacement arthroplasty.

Why is it reserved usually for people over fifty?

Because loosening or infection may occur after 10-15 years thus requiring revision — 15 years may see a lot of people out.

What two names are commonly associated with total replacement arthroplasty of the hip?

1. Charnley.
2. Muller.

Excision Arthroplasty

What is the other name for excision arthroplasty?

Girdlestone's pseudarthrosis.

In effect, what is Girdlestone's operation?

Excision of head and neck of femur and the upper half of the wall of the acetabulum.

What might be done with the gluteus medius muscle in this procedure?

It can be sutured into the gap thus created to act as a cushion between the bones.

Would you consider this procedure a salvage operation or primary operation?

A salvage operation. Girdlestone considered it a primary operation, but today it is usually reserved for failed total hip replacement.

Osteotomy

How does this work?

By displacing femoral shaft medially, pain relief is obtained by taking the weight off the damaged part of the femoral head.

Can it be converted to total hip replacement?

Yes.

Arthrodesis

What are the indications?

A painful arthritic hip in a young person with normal other hip (and normal knee on same side) and a painless back.

It is the only certain way of eliminating hip pain — true or false?

True.

CHAPTER 48

BURSAE ABOUT THE KNEE

* **Pre patellar bursitis.**
* Where is the pre patellar bursa situated? In front of the distal half of the patella and proximal part of the patellar tendon.

* Give two types of bursitis. Irritative and infective or suppurative.

* What is the other name for irritative pre patellar bursitis? Housemaid's Knee.

* As a result of repeated friction, what happens to the bursa? Fibrous thickening of the wall of the bursa occurs and it becomes filled with fluid.

Clinical Features

* Give two.
  1. Softly fluctuant swelling in front of the patella.
  2. The swelling is clearly demarcated.

* Give three possible ways of treating Housemaid's knee.
  1. Aspirate cyst under local anaesthetic and inject it with hydrocortisone.
  2. Excise the cyst.
  3. Avoid kneeling.

Infrapatellar Bursitis

Give its other name. Clergyman's Knee.

Locate it. Anterior to distal part of patellar tendon.

What is the treatment? Same as for Housemaid's Knee.

Semi-membranosus Bursa

Where is it located? Between the semi-membranosus and medial head of gastrocnemius behind the knee, medially.

How do you make it stand out? Straighten the knee.

Treatment? Excise it.

Can the fluid be pushed into the knee joint? No, because the muscles compress the opening.

Popliteal Cyst

Give its other name. Baker's Cyst.

Where is it located? Mid-line posteriorly, in the popliteal region.

Give two predisposing diseases.
1. Rheumatoid arthritis of the knee.
2. Osteoarthritis of the knee.

How is it treated? By aspiration and cortisone injection. Excision fails often because of underlying disease.

CHAPTER 49

CHONDROMALACIA PATELLAE

Define chondromalacia patellae.

Chondromalacia patellae is a painful condition of the knee seen in young persons and associated with pain and crepitus behind the kneecap, with flexion and extension movements.

Is it commoner in girls or boys?

Girls.

What is the commonest age group?

Adolescence.

What part of the patella is affected?

The cartilage of the articular surface becomes roughened and fibrillated.

Does chondromalacia patellae predispose to osteoarthritis at the patello-femoral joint?

Yes.

What is the aetiology of chondromalacia? Give three.

Uncertain.
1. Blow on patella.
2. Recurrent dislocation or subluxation.
3. Faulty line of movement of patella in flexion and extension.

An abnormally prominent ridge on the medial femoral condyle may or may not be responsible. Which is it?

May be responsible.

Clinical Features

Where is the pain located?

Behind the kneecap.

What makes the pain worse?

Walking up or down stairs or a slope.

Is effusion ever present?

Often it is present.

What is noted on displacing the patella from side to side?

This gives rise to pain.

Where else might there be well localized tenderness?

On the front of the medial femoral condyle.

What might be heard during movements of flexion and extension of the knee?

Fine crepitation can be felt and heard.

What do the radiographs usually show?

They are normal.

Treatment

Give three conservative methods of treatment.

1. Firm elastic bandage.
2. Restricted activities.
3. Isometric quadriceps exercises.

What might be done if symptoms persist?

Operation may be contemplated.

Name two operations that could be helpful.

Trimming of the prominent ridge on the front of the medial femoral condyle, or shaving posterior surface of patella.

Give another operation.

Medial transfer of the insertion of the patella tendon prevents recurrent dislocation of the patella and redirects its line of movement.

What might also be done by way of an operation on the lateral expansion of the quadriceps aponeurosis?

Release it, thus allowing medial shift of the patella.

Is there any place for patellectomy?

Yes, as a last resort.

CHAPTER 50

OSTEOCHONDRITIS DISSECANS OF THE KNEE

* Define osteochondritis dissecans of the knee.

Osteochondritis dissecans is an affliction of the knee in which a small area of the femoral condyle becomes necrotic causing pain and sometimes dislodging into the joint producing a loose body.

* What is the main pathology of this condition?

Local necrosis of the bone underlying a segment of articular cartilage.

* Name two possible fates of the necrotic bone with its overlying articular cartilage.

1. Eventual separation of the fragment with loose body formation.
2. Reunion of the necrotic bone in situ.

Does this condition take place in other joints?

Yes, but the knee is by far the most common joint affected.

What is the cause of osteochondritis dissecans of the knee?

Unknown — probably repeated minor trauma.

* What is a possible factor in causation?

Impairment of the blood supply to the affected segment of bone by thrombosis of an end artery.

Is injury a predisposing factor?

Yes.

Does it affect several joints in the one person?

Occasionally.

Is it sometimes familial?

Yes.

* What is the commonest part of the knee to be affected?

The articular surface of the medial condyle of the femur.

What is the usual size of the segment affected?

1-2 cubic centimetres.

At operation, what is noted about the overlying cartilage?

It is softer than normal articular cartilage.

What would histological examination of the subchondral bone show?

Avascularity.

* At operation, is there a clear line of demarcation between normal articular cartilage and the avascular segment?

Yes, it is very apparent.

How long after the onset of the condition does it take a loose body to form?

Several months.

What happens to the shallow cavity from which the loose body emerged?

It is ultimately filled with fibro cartilage.

The damage to the joint by having a cavity there may give rise to ..... later in life.

Osteoarthritis.

What is the usual age group for this condition?

Adolescence or young adult.

Clinical Features

* Give three typical symptoms.

1. Pain on exercise.
2. Feeling of insecurity in knee.
3. Intermittent swelling.

When loose body formation has taken place, what is the main symptom?

Recurrent locking episodes.

On physical examination, give four outstanding signs seen in osteochondritis dissecans of the knee.

1. An effusion is present.
2. Quadriceps muscle wasting.
3. Tender area on femoral condyle.
4. Loose body occasionally palpated.

* What may early radiographs reveal?

A clearcut defect on the articular surface of the medial femoral condyle.

What might be seen at a later date?

A loose body may be seen in the joint.

In what position does the radiograph show the defect most readily?

With a tangential postero-anterior projection with the knee semi-flexed.

Treatment

* In cases where loose body formation has not taken place, give two modes of treatment.

1. Support knee with crepe bandage.
2. Curtail strenuous activities.

* When the lesion is "ripe", i.e. when a clear line of demarcation is formed between the separating fragment and the surrounding normal bone, what treatment should be re-commended?

The loose piece should usually be removed leaving a small cavity.

What happens to the cavity?

Eventually it is filled with fibro cartilage.

* Under what circumstances should the displaced piece of bone be replaced into the femoral condyle?

When the piece of bone lying free in the joint is very large some surgeons like to replace it and hold it with a pin.

* Does this replacement of loose fragment always give rise to union?

Yes, usually it does.

* Does it always prevent osteoarthritis developing?

No.

CHAPTER 51

CONGENITAL CLUB FOOT

Define congenital club foot.

Congenital club foot is an inverting and plantar flexing deformity of the foot seen in affected infants at birth.

What is the other name for congenital club foot?

Talipes equino varus.

Why is club foot important?

Because it is the commonest congenital deformity of the foot.

What is the cause of club foot?

A defect of foetal development.

What part does intra uterine malposition of the foetal foot play in this condition?

Perhaps minor degrees of deformity may develop in this fashion.

Name two conditions that produce identical deformities in the foot.

1. Myelomeningocele.
2. Arthrogryposis.

Pathology

The soft tissues of the medial side of the foot are under-developed and ..... than normal.

Shorter.

In what position is the foot held? Give two.

1. It is adducted.
2. Inverted.

In what joints are these abnormalities noted? Give three.

1. Subtalar.
2. Mid tarsal and
3. Anterior tarsal joints.

In what position is the ankle held?

In equinus (plantar flexion).

What may happen to the calf and peroneal muscles?

They may be underdeveloped.

If untreated, what happens to the tarsal bones?

They become misshapen perpetuating the deformity.

Clinical Features

Is it commoner in boys or girls?

Commoner in boys.

Is congenital dislocation of the hip commoner in boys or girls?

Girls.

Does it affect one or both feet?

One or both. Bilateral in one third of cases.

What is the first feature noticed clinically?

When the infant is born, the foot is turned inwards so that the sole is directed medially.

What are the three elements of the deformity?

1. Inversion (twisting inwards) of the foot.
2. Adduction (inward deviation) of the forefoot relative to the hind foot.
3. Equinus (plantar flexion).

What is the main test that indicates the child has this malfunction of the foot?

The foot cannot be pushed passively through the normal range of eversion and dorsi flexion.

Diagnosis

What test should be applied to every baby to exclude congenital club foot?

The little toe should be able to be placed on the shin of the same side in any child under one year of age.

Prognosis

Upon which one factor does the prognosis depend?

The earlier the treatment the better the prognosis.

Primary Conservative Treatment

When should treatment begin?

Immediately after birth, certainly not more than one week later.

What are the principles of treatment? Name two.

1. To overcorrect the deformity by repeated manual pressure.
2. To hold the foot in the over corrected position until there is no longer a tendency for deformity.

In what order are the deformities corrected?

1. Adduction.
2. Inversion.
3. Equinus.

Is general anaesthesia used?

No.

How many manipulations might be necessary and at what intervals?

Six or eight manipulations at weekly intervals may be necessary.

Between manipulations, how might the correction be maintained?

By plaster of paris.
By metal splints (Denis Browne).

Of these two methods, which is preferred?

Plaster of paris because it is more efficient and lasts longer.

How high should the plaster extend?

To the upper thigh.

At what angle is the knee held?

Ninety degrees of flexion.

How often must the plaster be changed?

Once per week initially then it may be extended to two and then three weeks until the child grows larger.

With Denis Browne splints, how are the feet held?

Metal splints are strapped with adhesive strapping to the feet which are turned outwards.

How often should the splint be reapplied?

Every day.

At what point of time would you suggest operative treatment?

After three months if the feet are not normal clinically and radiologically.

What is the essence of the operation?

Release taut ligaments on the medial side of the ankle and foot and if need be, lengthen the calcaneal tendon.

For how long would you immobilize in plaster after this procedure?

Three months.

Treatment in Neglected or Relapsed Cases

What is the aim of treatment in neglected cases?

To produce a plantigrade foot which is equal to a foot with the sole on the ground.

How might this be achieved?

With repeated plaster of paris immobilizations after repeated manipulations.

If this should fail, what then?

Operative treatment is required.

Types of Operation

Children from 2-12 years.

Five operations are to be considered. What are they?

1. Division of short soft tissue on the medial side of the foot then plaster of paris immobilization.
2. Transfer of tendon of tibialis anterior lateral wards or tibialis posterior through the inter osseous membrane to the lateral side of the foot.
3. Lengthening of the short calcaneal tendon.
4. Arthrodesis of the calcaneo-cuboid joint with excision of a wafer of bone to shorten the lateral body of the foot.
5. When inversion of the heel is a prominent feature, osteotomy of the calcaneus with insertion of a bone wedge on the medial side to correct the line of weight bearing.

Children over twelve years.

The operations are directed to the bones after the age of twelve, because, before the age of twelve, growth of the foot might be disturbed. What is the operation over the age of twelve?

A wedge of bone of appropriate size based dorso-laterally is removed from the tarsus so that when the resulting gap is closed, the foot is plantigrade.

CHAPTER 52

* BUNION — HALLUX VALGUS

* Define bunion.

A bunion is a painful adventitious bursa overlying the medial exostosis of the first metatarsal in a patient with hallux valgus.

* Define hallux valgus.

Hallux valgus is a common female foot deformity in which the great toe is deviated laterally and associated with a painful exostosis and adventitious bursa formation at the medial side of the first metatarsal head.

* In hallux valgus, the great toe is deviated in which direction?

Laterally.

* At what joint is the deviation?

Metatarsophalangeal joint.

* In which sex is it commoner?

Women.

* In which age group, above or below middle-aged?

Above middle-aged.

Cause

* What forces push the toe laterally?

1. Tight stockings.
2. Pointed shoes.

What other aspect of the shoe probably aggravates the condition?

High heels force the foot down into the pointed end of the shoe.

Pathology

* The outstanding observation is that the big toe is deviated ..... and the first metatarsal is deviated in which direction?

Outward.
Medially.

* As a result of this latter abnormality, the gap between the heads of the first and second metatarsals is unduly ..... .

Wide.

What is the other name for the widening of this gap?

Metatarsus primus varus.

Is it possible on some occasions that this may be the primary defect?

Yes.

* Clinical Features

* Which sex is the commoner?

Female.

* What is the other name for the thick-walled bursa?

Bunion.

* In addition to osteoarthritis of the ..... joint, there is also ..... of the transverse arch.

Metatarsophalangeal.
Flattening.

* Is flattening of the transverse arch common or rare?

Common.

* On physical examination, the deformity of hallux valgus is obvious. The skin over the prominent joint has three features.

1. The skin is hard.
2. The skin is reddened.
3. The skin is tender.

* Sometimes the thick-walled bursa is filled with fluid.

* When secondary osteoarthritis has developed in the joint due to the malalignment, what happens to the movement? Give two features.

1. The movement is limited and
2. Painful.

* In later cases, the forefoot is not only flat and splayed but the other four toes manifest ..... .

Curling.

Treatment

* Give four conservative measures that may be used to give relief from hallux valgus.

1. Use wide footwear.
2. Regular chiropody.
3. Protection of bunion with pads.
4. Plastic wedge worn between great and second toe to reduce deformity.

* Give five possible operations that might be used for hallux valgus.

1. Keller's operation.
2. Mayo's operation.
3. Displacement osteotomy of the neck of the first metatarsal bone.
4. Arthrodesis of the metatarsophalangeal joint.
5. Trimming of exostosis.

* What does trimming of exostosis include?

Chiselling medial prominence off the metatarsal head.

* Is this operation recommended widely or not?

No, it frequently fails.

* In Keller's operation, what two structures are removed?

1. Excision of proximal half of proximal phalanx.
2. Excision of medial prominence of metatarsal head.

What happens to the space created between the proximal phalanx and the metatarsal head?

It is filled with fibrous tissue.

* Is Keller's operation a popular one?

Yes, extremely popular especially for the older age group.

The operation achieves four objectives. What are they?

1. It removes the painful bunion.
2. It corrects the deformity.
3. It creates a flail joint with increased passive movement.
4. It leaves a painless joint.

This operation known as Keller's operation leaves the great toe slightly ..... than normal and active movements of the toe are ..... .

Shorter.
Reduced.

What is Mayo's operation?

This includes excision of the first metatarsal head together with the sesamoid bones and bunion.

Is this operation common or rare?

Rare.

With regard to displacement osteotomy of the neck of the first metatarsal bone, after division of the neck, the head fragment is displaced in which direction?

Laterally (i.e. outwards).

How is the shaft fragment held to the head fragment? Give two methods.

1. By a spike of lateral cortex protruding from the shaft fragment and inserted into the head fragment.
2. By a screw or "K" wires.

Since the metatarsal head is shifted outwards, is it necessary to remove its medial prominence?

No.

The shifting of the head outwards also corrects the primary metatarsus varus.

As a result of course, the first and second metatarsal heads lie ....

Closer together.

In this operation, is the joint opened at all?

No.

After the operation, for how long would you immobilize the fragments in a plaster cast?

Eight weeks.

After this operation, is the toe shorter?

No.

After this operation, is there any impairment of active movement to the great toe?

No.

Since there is no loss of strength in the toe, it is very suitable for ..... people.

Young.

Arthrodesis: this leaves the patient with two toe features. What are they?

1. A painless joint.
2. A stiff metatarsophalangeal joint.

Is this operation popular?

No, because most people don't like the stiffness of the joint.

Generally speaking, the most popular operation is ..... in the older age group and metatarsal ..... in the younger.

Keller's; Osteotomy.

Basically the metatarsal osteotomy is designed to correct the .... and so realign the metatarsal and ....

Metatarsus primus varus.
Great toe.

CHAPTER 53

HAMMER TOE

* Define hammer toe.

Hammer toe is a painful condition in which there is a fixed flexion deformity of the proximal interphalangeal joint of the toe associated with callosity formation over that articulation.

* Which joint is involved in this deformity?

Proximal interphalangeal joint.

With hammer toe, is the flexion deformity of this joint fixed or mobile?

Fixed.

Cause

This is due to an imbalance of the delicate arrangement of ..... and ..... mechanisms.

Flexor; Extensor.

The precise reason for the defect is ..... .

Unknown.

Pathology

* The affected joint is sharply angled into ..... and contracture of the joint ..... on the plantar aspect has the effect of fixing the .....

Flexion.
Capsule.
Deformity.

* Usually something appears over the dorsum of the flexed joint. What is it?

A callosity.

Clinical Features

* Which is the commonest toe affected?

The second toe.

* It is characteristically seen that the proximal ..... joint is held in .... and the distal interphalangeal joint rests in ..... hyperextension.

Interphalangeal; Fixed flexion.
Compensatory.

What actually causes the pain with hammer toe?

The overlying callosity is painful.

Treatment

* Give four methods of treating hammer toe.

1. Do nothing.
2. Put a pad on the callosity.
3. Arthrodese the proximal interphalangeal joint in the straight position by using the pegging technique.
4. Proximal phalangectomy, either partial or complete.

CHAPTER 54

PAIN IN THE FOREFOOT

Is this common or rare?

Common.

Give another name for pain in the forefoot.

Metatarsalgia.

Give three causes of pain in the forefoot.

1. Anterior flat foot (dropped transverse arch).
2. Stress fracture of a metatarsal bone (March fracture).
3. Plantar digital neuroma (Morton's metatarsalgia).

Anterior Flat Foot

What is the other name for anterior flat foot?

Dropped transverse arch.

What is the commonest cause of metatarsalgia?

Anterior flat foot.

What is the cause of the pain in anterior flat foot?

Excessive weight bearing pressure beneath the metatarsal heads.

What is the primary cause of this condition?

Inefficiency of the intrinsic muscles of the foot.

In a normal situation, what effect does toe function have on the metatarsal heads?

The metatarsal heads can be raised from the ground by the action on the toes.

What muscles plantar flex the metatarsophalangeal joints? Give two.

The intrinsic muscles together with the long and short flexors.

In the normal foot, the weight is shared between what two structures in the forefoot?

1. The metatarsal heads.
2. The toes.

If the intrinsic muscles are inefficient, what happens to the toes?

They point upwards and don't share the weight bearing load of the metatarsal heads.

What effect does the excessive weight have on the ball of the foot?

Callosities develop.

Clinical Features

What is the main complaint?

Pain beneath the forefoot.

Give four findings on physical examination.

1. Forefoot is splayed.
2. Callosities beneath metatarsal heads.
3. Toes point upwards.
4. Patient unable to place toe tips on ground (indicating intrinsic muscle weakness).

Treatment of Anterior Flat Foot

What treatment would you recommend for a patient under fifty?

Physiotherapy to strengthen intrinsic muscles.

Name two operations that might be used if the pain is very severe.

1. Excision of head of metatarsal that is causing most of the discomfort (2nd metatarsal).
2. Osteotomy of neck of metatarsal and dorsal displacement of the head.

* Stress Fracture of a Metatarsal Bone

* Give two other names for this condition. — March fracture and fatigue fracture.

* Is there a history of violence with this fracture? — No.

* What is the cause of a march fracture? — Oft repeated and long continued stress as in taking a long walk on hard ground.

* Which metatarsals are usually involved? — Second or third metatarsal bones.

* Is the fracture ever displaced? — No. It is just a hairline fracture.

* If a swelling is felt at the fracture site, how does one explain this? — A large mass of callus forms a lump that is readily palpable.

* What is the main complaint? — Pain in forefoot on walking.

* Give two features on physical examination. — Swelling on top of forefoot plus well-localized tenderness.

* Give two radiographic findings. —
  1. Hairline crack early on.
  2. Callus formation seen three weeks post symptom onset.

Treatment

* How is this treated? — The fracture always heals so simply recommend reduced activity or if pain is very intense below knee walking plaster with a heel.

Morton's Metatarsalgia

* Give two other names for this condition. —
  1. Plantar digital neuritis.
  2. Inter digital neuroma.

Pathology

* What happens to the digital nerve? — Fibrous thickening or neuroma formation takes place where the nerve lies between metatarsal heads.

Which digital nerve is commonly involved? — The one between the third and fourth cleft.

What part of the nerve is involved? — The neuroma forms immediately proximal to the point of division into terminal branches of the nerve.

How long is the fusiform swelling in the nerve? — About one centimetre.

What is the cause of the fibrous thickening? — Unknown.

Is it commoner in men or women? — Women.

Is it the younger age group or middle age? — Middle age.

* When does the pain occur? — On standing or walking.

* Whence does the pain radiate? — To the contiguous sides of the third and fourth toes.

What classically relieves the pain? — Taking the shoe off and squeezing or manipulating the foot.

* Give two forms of treatment.

Sponge rubber metatarsal pad may help. Should the metatarsal pad fail, operative excision of the thickened segment of nerve is recommended.

* Plantar Wart

Give two other names for this condition.

1. Verruca pedis.
2. Verruca plantaris.

* Where do plantar warts occur in the sole of the foot?

Anywhere.

* How do they differ from warts elsewhere?

Warts on other parts of the body project beyond the skin surface, whereas plantar warts are flush with the skin.

* How do they differ from plantar callosities?

A plantar callosity develops only at a point of pressure as under a metatarsal head.

What is the cause of plantar wart?

Probably a viral infection.

* What is a wart?

A simple papilloma growing outwards from the basal layers of the skin.

What happens to the skin surrounding the wart?

It is thickened and raised.

Is there a line of demarcation between the wart and the surrounding thickened skin?

Yes.

How is this tiny cleft visualized?

By stretching the skin away from the wart.

* Give two ways of treating this condition.

Apply caustics in the first instance and if this fails, cauterize the base of the wart.

* Callosities

* What is a callosity?

A localized thickening of the skin in response to abnormal pressure.

* Where do plantar callosities occur?

Under prominent bones, e.g. metatarsal heads.

* Whereabouts do callosities occur on toes?

On the dorsum of the toe that is unduly prominent or on the tip of a flexed hammer toe.

* What is the other name for a callosity on a toe?

A corn.

* How do you treat this condition?

By removing the underlying bone causing the pressure.

Give two other ways of treating this condition.

1. Removing excess epidermis.
2. Sponge rubber padding over the thickened area.

CHAPTER 55

EXAMINATION OF THE HIP JOINT

* Before we examine the hip joint, we enquire about the patient's symptoms. What are the four common symptoms associated with hip disorders?

1. Pain.
2. Limp.
3. Stiffness.
4. Shortening.

* Is the pain in the front or the back of the hip joint usually?

Usually the front.

* If the pain radiates, does it go upward or downward?

Usually down the front of the thigh toward the knee.

* When we examine any joint, we follow the drill of ....., ... , ... , ...

Inspection, Palpation, Movement, X-ray.

* What do we seek on inspecting the skin? Give two.

1. Scars.
2. Sinuses.

* What do we seek with regard to the shape of the hip area? Give three.

1. Asymmetry.
2. Swelling.
3. Wasting.

* What do we look for with regard to joint position? Give two.

1. Deformity.
2. Shortening.

* When we are feeling the joint area passing from superficial to deep, the first level palpated is the ..... .

Skin.

* The second level we feel are the ....

Soft tissues.

* The third feature we seek is the ....

Bone structure.

* Little is detected with regard to the palpation of skin and soft tissues about the hip joint, but when it comes to feeling the bones we can estimate the position of the head of the femur.

* When feeling for the head of the femur initially, where are the thumbs placed?

On the anterior, superior iliac spines.

* On what bony prominence are the middle fingers placed?

On the greater trochanters.

* From the above position the thumbs are then moved ..... in an attempt to feel the head of the femur. If the head is not in the socket, the thumb sinks in too far.

Medially.

* Enumerate the movements of the hip joint. Give six.

1. Flexion.
2. Extension.
3. Abduction.
4. Adduction.
5. Internal Rotation.
6. External Rotation.

* In what position do you place the patient to test for extension of the hip joint?

Face down (prone).

* All other hip joint movements are tested with the patient ..... .

Supine.

* What is the normal range of extension at the hip joint?

Approximately thirty degrees.

* Test yourself also for the range of flexion at the hip joint and see what it is.

Approximately one hundred and forty degrees.

* The movements of abduction and adduction are demonstrated. In testing abduction, the leg being tested is moved .... the mid line.

Away from.

* In testing adductoin, the leg being tested is moved across the ....

Other leg.

* What are the two types of rotation at the hip joint that must be tested?

Internal and external.

* When testing internal rotation, the foot is turned ..... .

Inwards.

* When testing external rotation, the foot is turned ..... .

Outwards.

* When testing the rotational movements, what bone is used as an index of the degree of rotation?

The patella.

* In considering the shortening of the limb, we talk about two types of shortening. What are they?

Real and apparent.

* What is meant by real shortening?

Real shortening means that the leg is actually short and can be measured to be short.

* What is meant by apparent shortening?

With apparent shortening, there is a tilt in the pelvis giving the impression that one leg is shorter than the other but measurements, of course, show this may not be the case.

* When measuring real shortening, what two points are used?

The distance between the anterior, superior, iliac spine and the tip of the medial malleolus is measured with the knee straight, and the pelvis at right angles to the long axis of the body.

* When examining the hip with the patient lying on his face, we look for ....., ... or .....

Scars, Sinuses, Wasting.

* When examining the patient lying on his face, we feel and look for ....

Muscle bulk.

* When examining the patient lying on his face, we test a particular movement and compare it with a similar movement of the other hip. What is that movement?

Extension of the hips are best treated with the patient lying on his face.

* Trendelenburg's sign. When the normal person stands on one leg, the opposite hip ..... .

Rises.

* This can be tested yourself by standing with your hands on your iliac crests. If, when you stand on one leg, the opposite hip falls, this is known as a positive ....

Trendelenburg's sign.

* When the normal person stands on one foot, the opposite hip is elevated because of the pull of which muscles? Give two.

1. Gluteus medius   ) on the weight bearing
2. Gluteus minimus)   side of the body.

* If these two muscles are weak or inflamed or have a defective fulcrum through which to work, the pelvis cannot be tilted and as a result, we have a positive ....

Trendelenburg's sign.

* Give four causes for a positive Trendelenburg's sign.

1. Weak gluteus medius and gluteus minimus muscles due to poliomyelitis.
2. Inflammation of the above muscles.
3. Fractured neck of femur.
4. Congenital dislocation of the hip joint.

Radiographs

* In viewing the radiographs of the hip joint, look at the picture as a whole and observe the ....

Bone density.

* After that, observe the joint itself with special reference to the joint space. This may be ..... or ..... .

Decreased; Increased.

* Also observe the joint line to see if it is ..... .   Eroded.

* If the joint space is decreased, one would expect ..... .

Osteoarthritis.

* If the joint space is increased, one would expect ....

An effusion. (Fluid in the joint produces widening of the joint space.)

CHAPTER 56

EXAMINATION OF THE KNEE JOINT

* When examining a knee joint, it is essential to compare one knee with ....

The other.

* It is best, therefore, if the patient removes his ....., ... and ..... .

Trousers, shoes, socks.

Symptoms

* Enumerate the common symptoms pertaining to disorders of the knee joint. Give six.

1. Pain.
2. Swelling.
3. Locking.
4. Clicking.
5. Giving way.
6. Limping.

Physical Examination of the Knee Joint

* What are the common headings under which we examine any joint? Give four.

1. Inspection.
2. Palpation.
3. Movement.
4. Radiographs.

* What are the precise points you observe when inspecting the knee? Give three.

1. Skin.
2. Shape.
3. Position.

* What might be observed on inspection of the skin about the knee? Give three.

1. Colour of the skin.
2. Presence of sinuses.
3. Presence of scars.

* With regard to shape, one would observe on looking perhaps two features. What might they be?

1. Swelling of the knee.
2. Wasting of the muscles (quadriceps).

* In which abnormal position might you find the knee? Give four.

1. Flexed.
2. Hyperextended.
3. Valgus.
4. Varus.

* When it comes to palpation or feeling the joint, we move from superficial to deep and, therefore, feel firstly the ....., secondly .... and thirdly ..... .

Skin; Soft tissues. Bones.

* When palpating the skin, we usually look for ....

Temperature variations.

* If, for example, the skin of the knee feels hot, then one would expect an inflammatory condition of the knee joint. When feeling the soft tissues, we test for ..... .

Fluid.

* Fluid in the knee lifts the patella away from the femoral condyles. When the patella is tapped, it can be felt to strike against the femoral condyles and this test for fluid in the knee is known as the ....

Patella tap test.

* When there is no fluid in the knee as is the normal situation, the patella is in contact with the femoral condyles and the patella tap sign is then said to be ..... .

Negative.

* How else may one test a knee for presence of fluid?

By cross fluctuation test.

* When feeling the soft tissues about the knee, we must look just above the knee to the ..... muscle.

Quadriceps.

* This muscle should be felt and measured on both sides to see if there be any ..... .

Wasting.

* When palpating the bones about the knee, in what position is the knee held?

In ninety degrees of flexion.

* List the various parts that ought to be felt so far as the bony structure of the knee is concerned. Give five.

1. Femoral condyles.
2. Tibial condyles.
3. Joint lines — medial.
4. Joint lines — lateral.
5. The attachments of the ligaments must also be palpated.

* When testing the movements of the knee joint, we seek seven movements. What are they?

1. Flexion.
2. Extension.
3. Abduction.
4. Adduction.
5. Rotation.
6. Antero-posterior glide.
7. Retro-patellar movements.

* How far does the normal knee flex?

Till the calf meets the thigh muscle.

* The normal knee extends completely with a ..... .

Snap.

* The movements of abduction and adduction at the knee are normally ..... .

Zero.

* These movements would be present if there were any laxity of the medial or lateral ..... .

Ligaments.

* When testing for rotation, the tibial condyles are rotated on the femoral condyles with the knee flexed to ....

Ninety degrees.

* The specific rotation test which may be diagnostic for a torn meniscus is known as the ..... test.

McMurray.

* In McMurray's test, the ..... is rotated in almost full ..... .

Knee.
Flexion.

* While this is being performed, the knee is subjected to an ..... force.

Abduction.

* What is observed with a positive McMurray sign that may mean the patient has a torn meniscus?

The rotation of the tibial condyles on the femoral condyles as described above may produce pain or a click or the cartilage may actually be felt to protrude.

* When testing for antero-posterior glide, the patient's hips are flexed ..... degrees and his knees ..... degrees. The surgeon then steadies the limbs by ..... on the patient's feet. Using both hands, an attempt is made to move the ..... backwards and forwards on the ....

Forty-five.
Ninety.
Sitting.

Tibia; Femoral condyles.

* Moving the patella about from side to side on the femoral condyles produces a grating sensation in that condition known as ..... .

Osteoarthritis.

* Examination of the knee is not complete until the patient has been examined whilst lying on his face. We look in the popliteal region for .... and ..... .
We feel in this popliteal region for ..... .

Scars; Swellings.
Lumps.

Give two special investigations used to observe the internal anatomy of the knee.

1. Arthrogram.
2. Arthroscopic examination.

PICTORIAL SECTION
Including Explanations

The black and white prints 20–28 inclusive have been reproduced from 'A Colour Atlas of Hand Conditions' by kind permission of the author W. Bruce Conolly and the publishing firm, Wolfe Medical Publications Ltd. London.

The black and white prints 20-28 inclusive have been reproduced from 'A Colour Atlas of Hand Conditions' by kind permission of the author W. Bruce Conolly and publisher Wolfe Medical Publications Ltd., London.

PICTURES AND EXPLANATIONS

Pictures are not necessarily in numerical order.

1. A-P and lateral views of Colles' fracture in a child — note the presence of the epiphyses at the distal end of radius and ulna. There is marked dorsal and radial displacement of the distal fragments.

2. A-P view of fractures of both bones of forearm in a child. The presence of the epiphyses at the distal end of radius and ulna indicates the patient's youthfulness.

3. A-P and lateral views of Colles' fracture with dorsal displacement of the distal fragment as seen in the right hand picture — before closure of epiphyses.

4. Crack fracture of mid section of 5th metacarpal shaft.

5. A-P and lateral views of wrist depicting fractures in the lower third of both bones. Note the dorsal and ulna deviation of the smaller distal fragments.

6. Three views of healing fractures of lower radius and ulna. The dorsal angulation is of little consequence in a young person because moulding will straighten the bones ultimately.

7. A-P view of a normal wrist in a child. A child? Yes, because epiphyses are present.

8. Lateral view of Colles' fracture.

9. A-P view of normal wrist in an adult.

10. A-P view of Colles' fracture showing union of radial fragment and non union of ulna styloid.

11. Three views of wrist joint showing healed Colles' fracture with some mal-union. Note osteoarthritis at carpo-metacarpal joint — a coincidental finding.

12. Healing fracture of base of first metacarpal bone. This is not a Bennett's fracture since it does not involve the carpo-metacarpal joint.

13. A-P view of wrist showing fracture of scaphoid.

14. Two views of wrist joint depicting fracture of scaphoid.

15. A-P view of the three phalanges of middle finger — the proximal phalanx demonstrating an enchondroma.

16. Proximal phalanx of finger showing enchondroma.

16b. Enchondroma of proximal phalanx of fingers. The phalanx has fractured through the enchondroma.

17. Here we see the Galeazzi fracture dislocation. There is a combination of fracture of the shaft of the radius with dislocation of the inferior radio-ulna joint.

18. A-P view demonstrating Greenstick fracture of lower radius.

19. A-P view of carpal bones, showing fracture of base of first metacarpal. In the case of a Bennett's fracture there is involvement of the nearby carpo-metacarpal joint and that is not the case here.

20. Print showing ganglion on volar aspect of radial side of wrist.

21. A print showing the common position of a ganglion on the dorsal aspect of the wrist.

22. This picture demonstrates wrist drop. The patient sustained an injury to the radial nerve above the elbow. There is an inability to extend the wrist, fingers and thumb due to the paralysis of those dorsi flexing muscles supplied by the radial nerve.

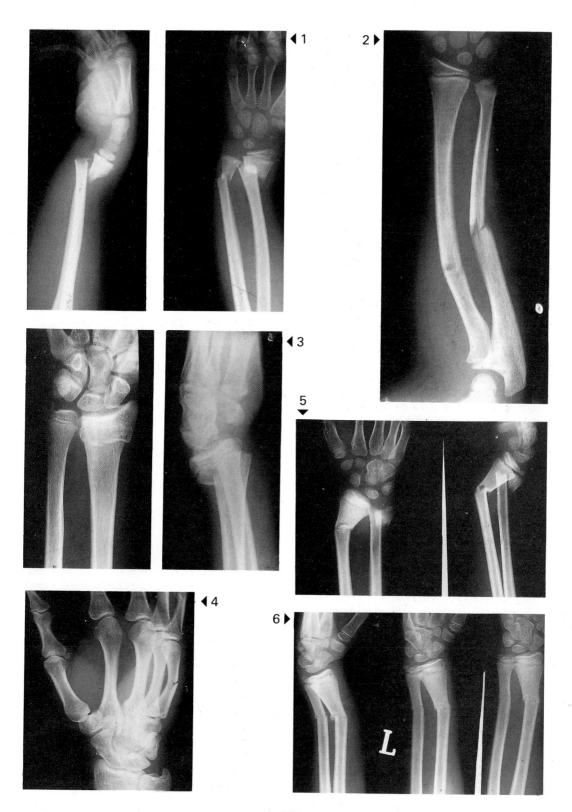

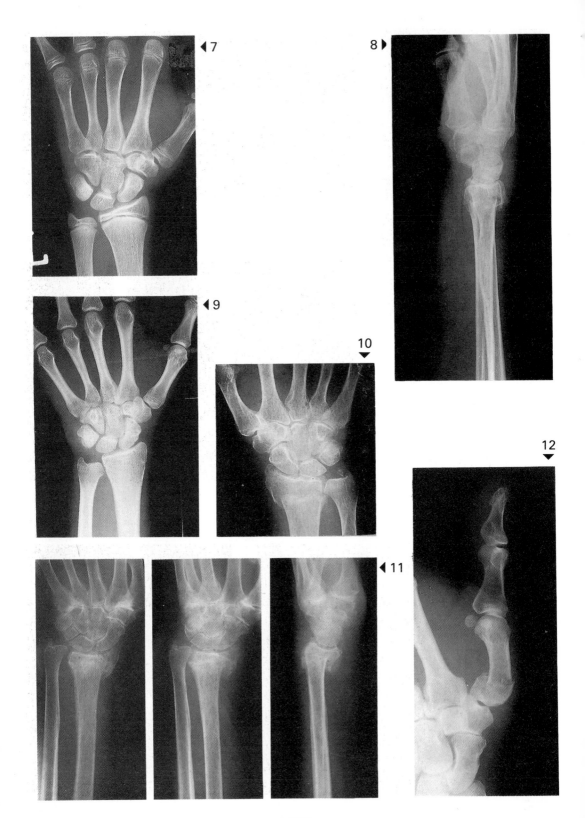

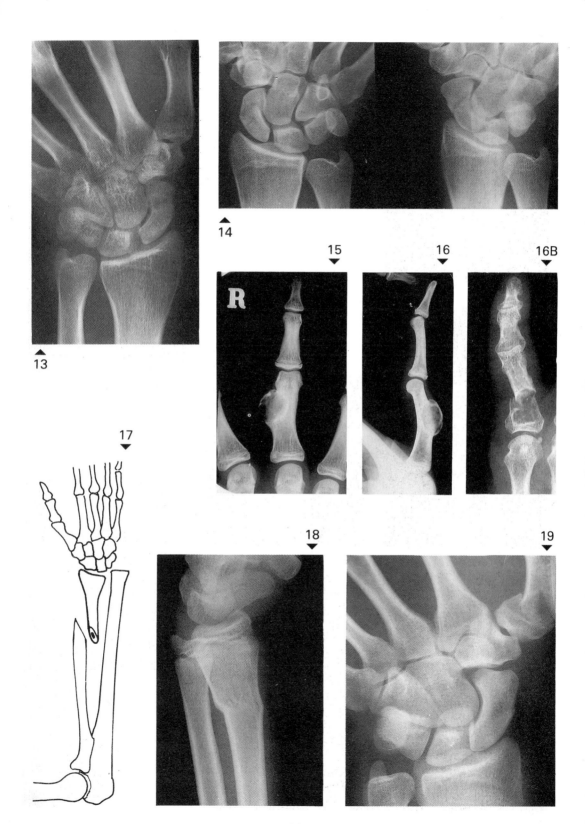

13

14

15

16

16B

17

18

19

231

23. Print showing laceration of ulna nerve at the wrist and the resulting intrinsic paralysis prevents flexion of the metacarpo-phalangeal and interphalangeal joints of ring and little fingers.

24. These hands demonstrate Dupuytren's contracture – the contracture of the palmar fascial bands produces flexion contracture of the metacarpo-phalangeal and proximal interphalangeal joints. Here we see involvement of the left little and right middle finger.

25. Picture of left hand demonstrating Dupuytren's contracture of left little finger.

26. These hands demonstrate rheumatoid arthritis of the metacarpophalangeal joints demonstrating the ulna deviation and proliferative synovitis.

27. Here we see a median nerve injury at the wrist. Note the area of sensory loss that usually includes the radial half of the ring finger as well as the middle, index and thumb areas.

28. This print demonstrates a mallet finger with closed rupture of the terminal extensor tendon following a crush injury.

The black and white prints 20-28 inclusive have been reproduced from 'A Colour Atlas of Hand Conditions' by kind permission of the author W. Bruce Conolly and publisher Wolfe Medical Publications Ltd., London.

29. A-P view of a normal elbow.

30. Lateral view of a normal elbow.

31. A-P view of child's elbow showing fracture of neck of radius – note the presence of the epiphyses indicating the approximate age of patient.

32. Lateral view of elbow showing a Monteggia fracture. Note the forward displacement of head of radius and ventral angulation of fracture of ulna.

33. Lateral view of fractured olecranon process.

34. Lateral view of dislocated elbow.

35. A-P view of elbow depicting fracture of neck of radius with slight displacement.

36. Lateral view of elbow showing supra-condylar fracture of lower humerus.

37. Lateral view of elbow and forearm depicting Paget's disease of radius. Note the upper radius is thick and bent.

38. A-P view of lower half of humerus demonstrating osteosarcoma of that bone. Note the elevation of periosteum forming the Codman's triangle and the sunray effect, also, lysis of the lower humerus can be seen.

39. A-P view of a normal elbow.

40. A-P view of a forearm demonstrating Paget's disease of the radius. Note that the radius is thick and bent and has areas of increased and decreased density.

41. A-P view of the wrist showing Colles' fracture undisplaced. Note the crack in the radius and ulna styloid.

42. A-P radiograph of humerus demonstrating mal-union in a transverse fracture of the upper third of the humerus with shortening of the bone and overriding with a small amount of callus formation.

43. A-P view of wrist area demonstrating fracture of tuberosity of scaphoid – undisplaced.

44. A-P view of normal shoulder.

45. A-P view of shoulder showing calcification of supra spinatus tendon.

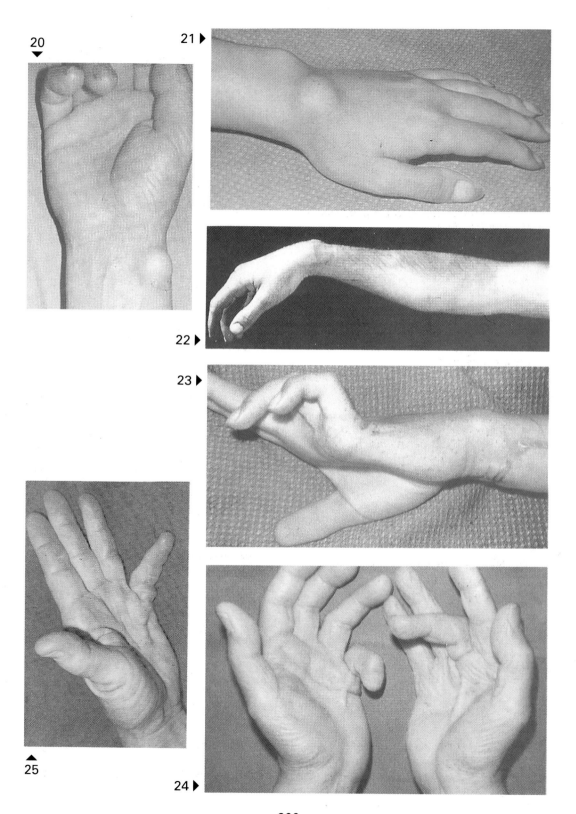

20

21 ▶

22 ▶

23 ▶

24 ▶

25 ▲

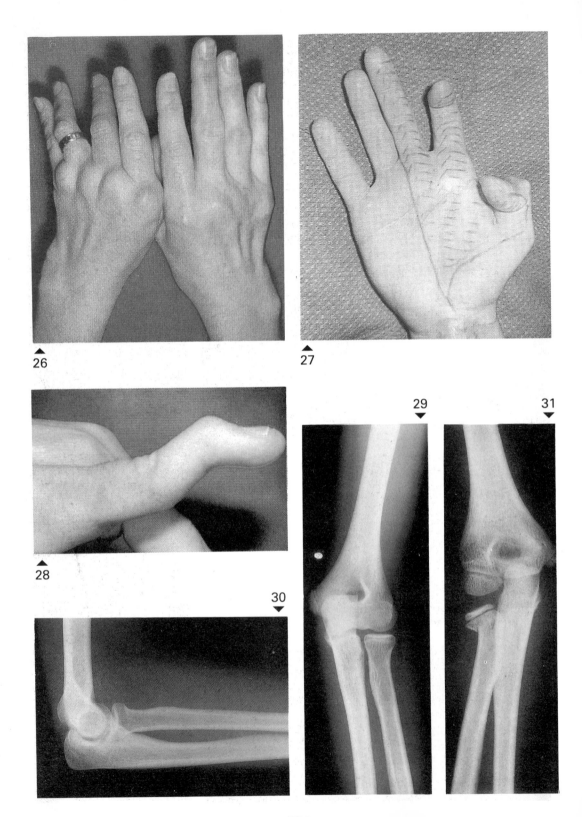

26

27

28

29

30

31

234

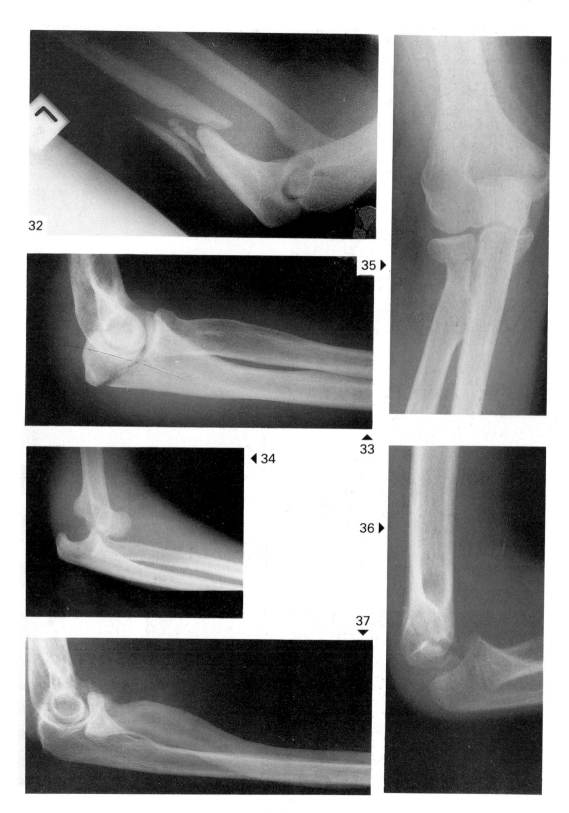

32

35 ▶

33
▲

◀ 34

36 ▶

37
▼

46. A-P view of the shoulder showing sub-coracoid dislocation of the upper humerus.

47. A-P view of upper humerus demonstrating fracture of the upper shaft of that bone in a child. Note the presence of the epiphysis of upper end of humerus.

48. A-P view of the shoulder demonstrating sub-coracoid dislocation of the upper humerus.

49. A-P view of left shoulder demonstrating fracture of outer third of clavicle.

50. A-P view of upper cervical spine taken through the mouth, depicting fracture of the dens or odontoid process of the axis.

51. A-P view of upper cervical spine showing a normal intact odontoid process once again filmed through the mouth.

52. A-P view through the mouth showing normal axis with intact dens or odontoid process.

53. A-P view taken through the mouth and showing fracture of dens or odontoid process.

54. Lateral radiograph of the skull demonstrating deposits of multiple myeloma – note punched out appearance of these many defects in the skull.

55. Lateral view of normal cervical spine.

56. A-P view of fracture in outer third of clavicle.

57. A-P view of upper thorax depicting oblique fracture in lateral third of clavicle.

58. A-P view of an united fracture of mid section of humerus.

59. A-P view of normal upper humerus.

60. A-P view demonstrating thoraco-lumbar scoliosis.

61. A-P view of lumbar spine demonstrating the bamboo spine associated with ankylosing spondylitis.

62. Lateral radiograph of lower lumbar spine depicting L–4 and L–5 vertebral bodies and the first sacral body. A discogram has been performed at L–4–5 and this indicates an L–4–5 disc protrusion because the radio opaque material passes posteriorly as far as the posterior vertebral border so one concludes the annulus must be bulging into the spinal canal to permit ths. At L–5.S–1 the discogram is said to be normal and it demonstrates the clear area above the dye, being the cartilage plate separating the dye from L–5 vertebral body and the clear area below the dye indicating the cartilage plate separating the dye from the superior surface of the first sacral body.

63. Lateral view of lumbar spine demonstrating a myelogram with indentation of the Myodil column due to an L–4–5 disc prolapse.

64. Lateral view of lumbar spine demonstrating a normal lumbar myelogram.

65. C.T. scan demonstrating prolapsed disc compressing the thecal sac marked "D".

66. A normal C.T. scan of lumbar spine. V is the vertebral body, T is the thecal sac which contains the cauda equina and S is the spinous process.

67. Demonstrates a C.T. scan with a sequestrated disc impinging on the thecal sac on the right side.

68. A-P view of a normal hip joint.

69. A lateral view of a normal hip joint.

70. A-P view showing congenital dislocation of the left hip. Note the absence of upper femoral capital epiphysis and exaggerated sloping of the left acetabulum as well as the lateral displacement of the upper shaft of femur.

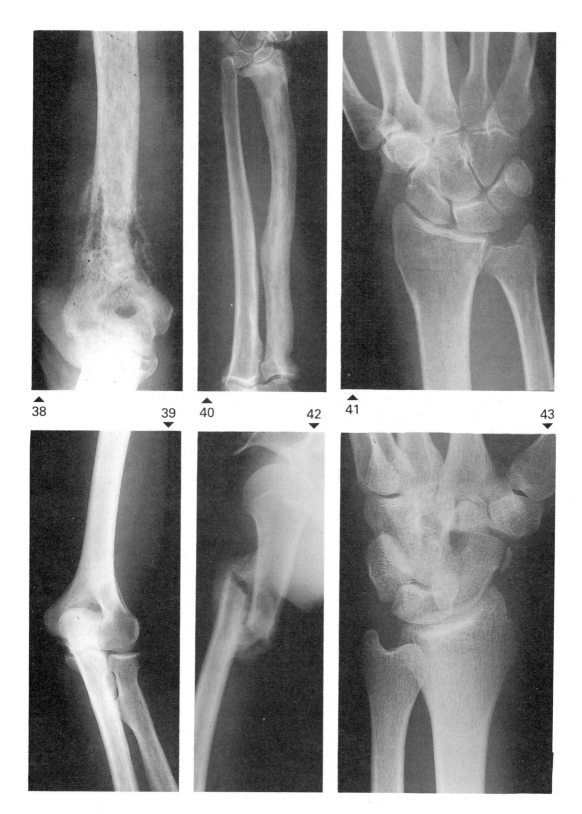

38

39

40

42

41

43

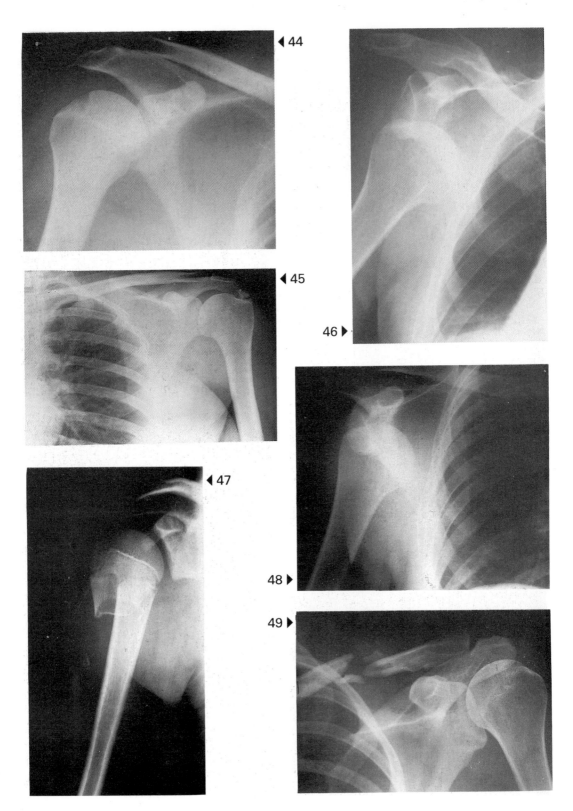

44

45

46 ▶

47

48 ▶

49 ▶

238

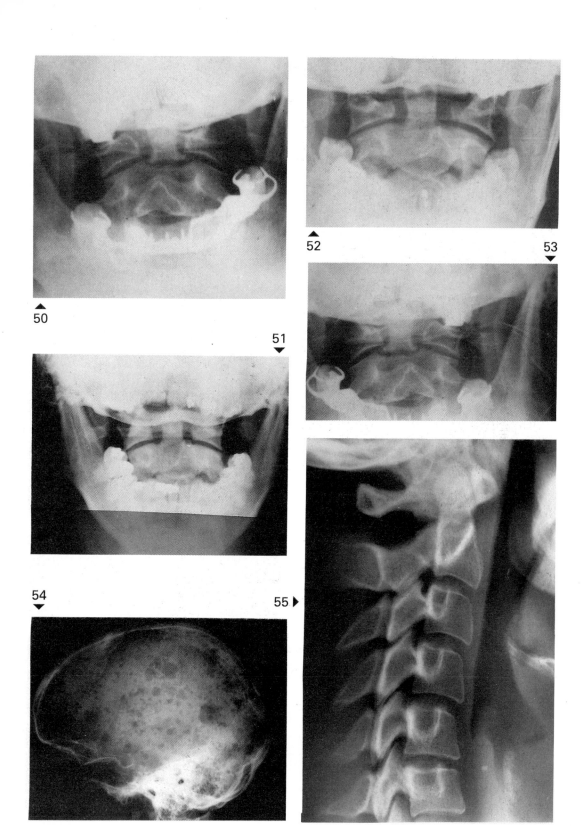

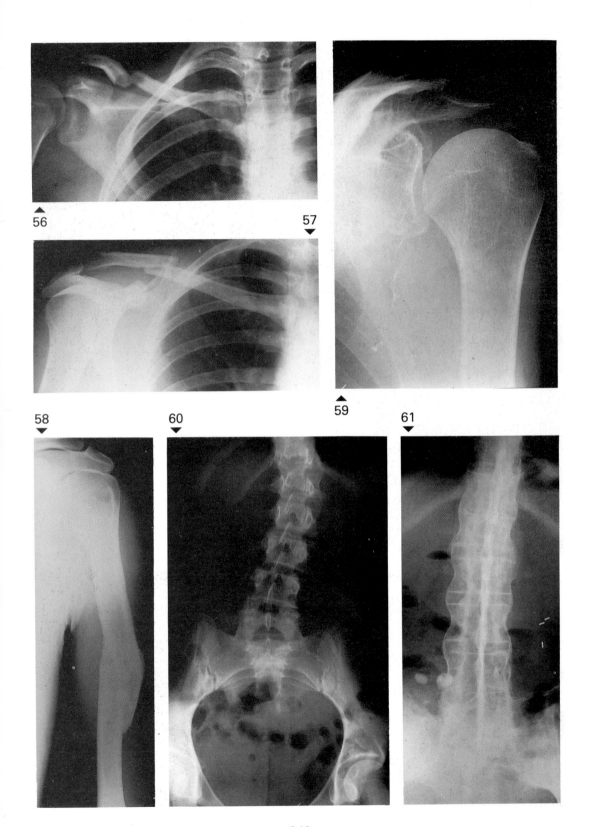

56

57

58

59

60

61

240

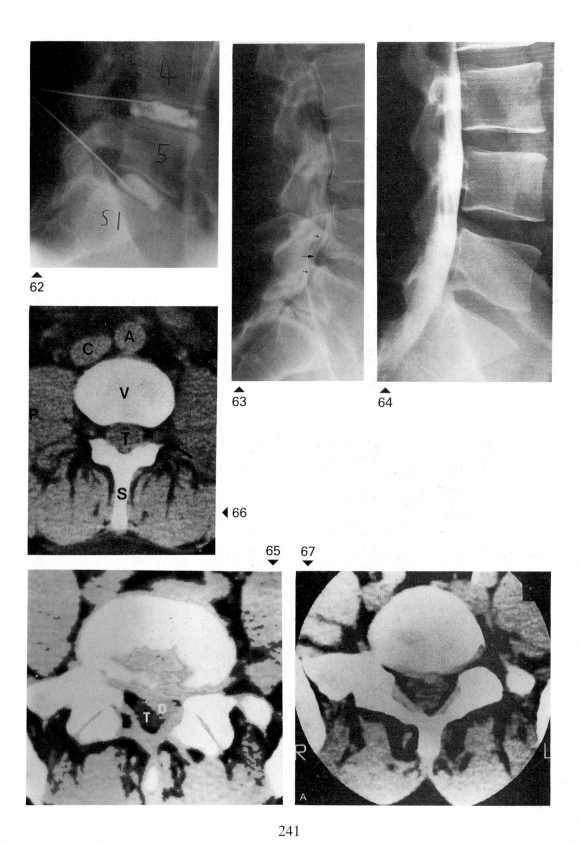

▲
62

▲
63

▲
64

◀66

65   67
▼   ▼

241

71. A-P view of pelvis demonstrating congenital dislocation of the right hip joint. Note the absence of the ossific centre of the involved side and the lateral and upward displacement of the upper femur together with the sloping nature of the acetabulum on the involved side. The pelvis on the involved side is smaller than its fellow.

72. A-P view demonstrating bilateral congenital dislocation of the hip.

73. A-P view showing osteoarthritis of the hip joint. Note the thin and irregular joint line and joint space and cyst formation with sclerosis of bone and exostosis formation.

74. A-P view of a pertrochanteric fracture of upper femur held in the correct position with a one piece Jewett pin and plate and four screws.

75. Fractured neck of femur held rigidly with a sliding compression screw and plate and four screws. This fixation device may be used for mid cervical or basilar fractures of neck of femur.

76. A-P view demonstrating fractures of each neck of femur. One is held with a sliding compression screw as seen on the right femur and the other with a pin plate and multiple screws.

77. A-P view of fractured neck of femur in a child.

78. Lateral view of hip joint showing Perthe's disease. Note the whitened vascular flattened upper femoral epiphysis. The whiteness implies avascularity.

79. A-P view of pelvis demonstrating severe osteoarthritis of the right hip and a replacement prosthesis has been applied to relieve the pain of the arthritis of the opposite hip.

80. Sub-capital fracture of the neck of femur in an osteoarthritic hip.

81. The pathology demonstrated in picture 80 has been treated with a Charnley's total hip replacement operation.

82. This A-P picture demonstrates a Thompson's prosthesis replacing the head of the femur that had manifested a sub-capital fracture.

83. A-P view of a basal fracture of neck of femur treated with Thornton pin and plate and screws. Note the screw lengths are such that they engage the medial cortex thus giving added strength.

84. A-P radiograph depicting posterior dislocation of hip joint.

85. A-P radiograph of the hip joint demonstrating gross osteoarthritis. Note the sclerosis of acetabulum and head of femur adjacent to the acetabulum and the obliteration of the joint space and irregularity of the joint line.

86. A-P view of pelvis showing unilateral Perthe's disease on the left side with flattening of the upper epiphysis of femur thus producing an increase in the joint space and the white appearance of the epiphysis indicates avascularity.

87. A-P view of pelvis and upper femora indicating Paget's disease.

88. A-P radiograph of pelvis indicating a right sided total hip replacement that has gone on to dislocation of the femoral component.

89. A-P radiograph of hip joint that has undergone replacement of femoral component with a Moore's prosthesis. This prosthesis is used commonly for fracture of the sub-capital type of neck of femur in elderly women. Note the three windows or fenestra that distinguish the Moore's from the Thompson prostheses. Through these windows may be passed cancellous bone derived from the head of the femur and this acts as a bone graft that locks the Moore's prosthesis into position permanently.

90. A-P view of hip joint demonstrating central dislocation of femoral head.

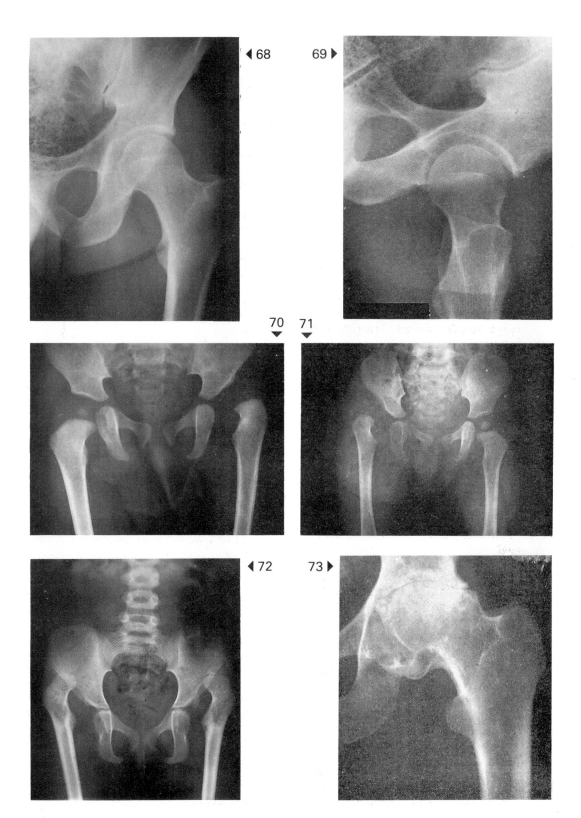

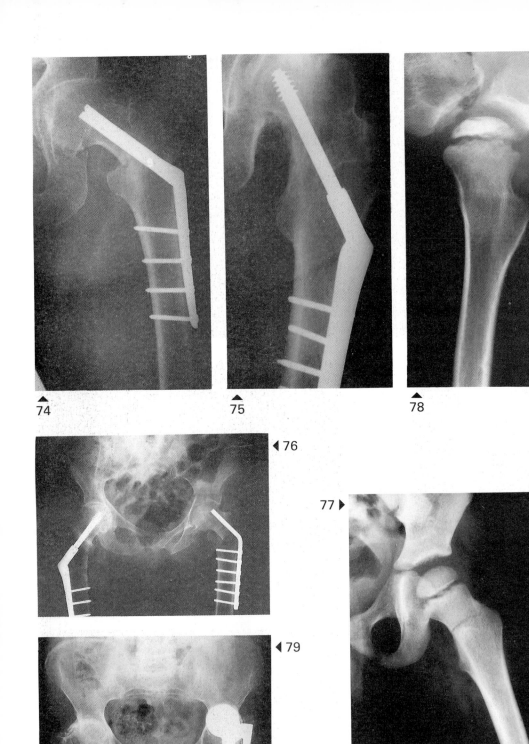

74   75   78

◄76

77▶

◄79

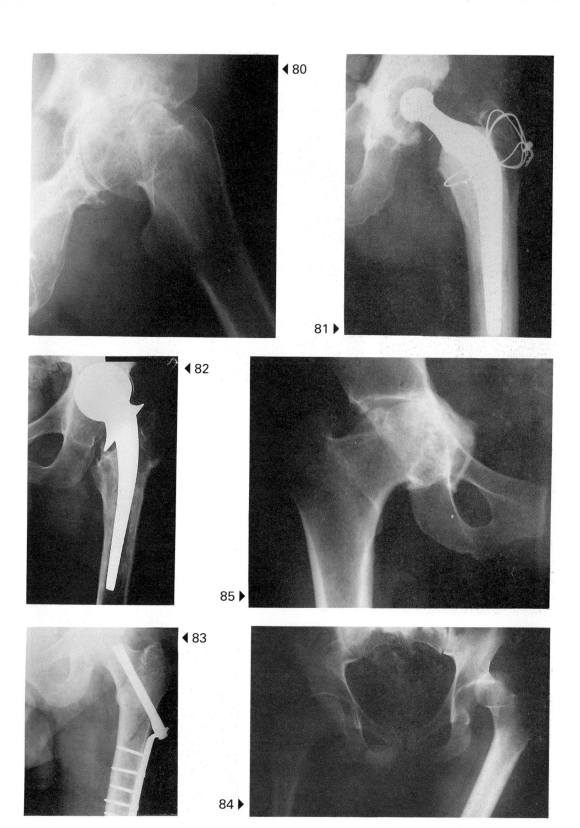

◀ 80

81 ▶

◀ 82

85 ▶

◀ 83

84 ▶

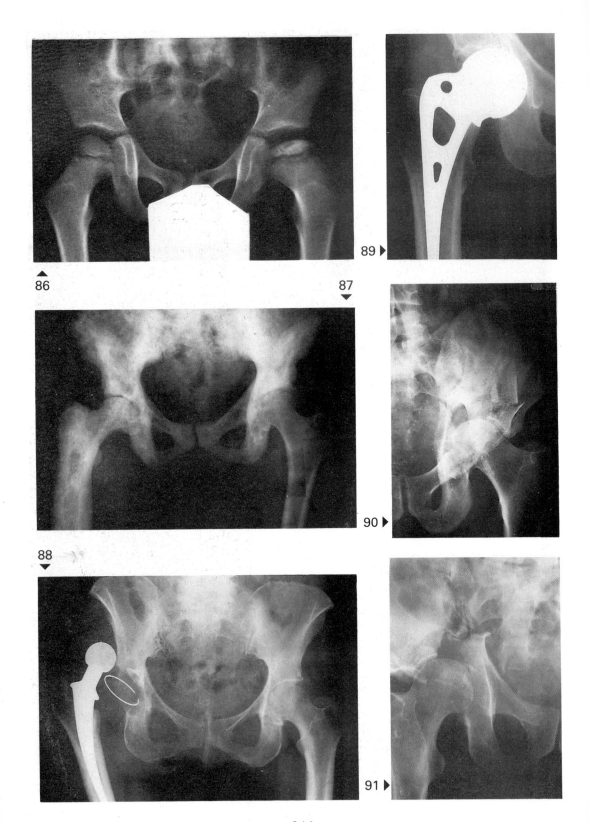

86

87

88

89 ▶

90 ▶

91 ▶

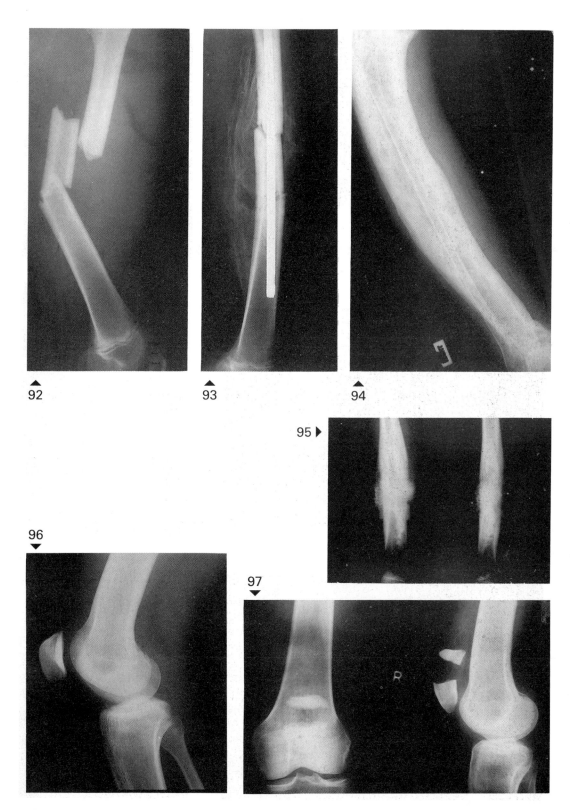

92

93

94

95 ▶

96

97

91. A-P radiograph of hip joint indicating central dislocation of femoral head.

92. Radiograph indicating fracture of the shaft of the femur in two places giving rise to three segments.

93. Kuntschner nail used to immobilize the fragments depicted in print 92.

94. Paget's disease of the tibia. Typically a hot thick bent bone (also shows relatively normal fibula).

95. Radiograph of femur depicting osteosarcoma – note the sunray effect.

96. Lateral view of normal knee joint.

97. A-P and lateral views of knee joint manifesting avulsion fracture of patella as seen in both views.

98. A-P and lateral view of knee joint showing avulsion fracture of patella.

99. Lateral view of normal knee in a child.

100. A-P view of hip joints demonstrating a slip of the upper right femoral epiphysis. A line passing upward along the superior border of the neck of the femur does not pass through the epiphysis as it should do in a normal hip joint, the reason for this being that the epiphysis has slipped.

101. A-P view of pelvis and femora demonstrating myelomatosis. Note the multiple myeloma deposits giving rise to areas of rarefaction.

102. Lateral radiograph showing a transverse fracture of the pathological type in the lower third of the femur – the bone is dense and has lost its medullary cavity.

103. Radiograph of the femur showing a sarcoma. Note the sunray effect of bony spicules and elevation of the periosteum giving rise to Codman's triangle. Also note the increased density of the bone.

104. Radiograph of the lower two thirds of femur in a lateral view indicating a Ewing's tumour. Note the osteolytic area in the centre of the femur rather than in the metaphyses region where most tumours arise.

105. Radiograph of a femur showing Paget's disease. Note the thickening of one cortex on the concave side and the bowing of the femur and the lack of density on the convex side due to increased blood supply to that part.

106. A-P radiograph of the knee showing chronic osteomyelitis of lower femur together with osteoarthritis of the knee joint itself. In the lower third of the femur one can see areas of rarefaction and the cortex and medulla merge. There is also increased density and sclerosis of the lower third of the femur.

107. Lateral radiograph of a knee joint that has undergone total replacement. The curved upper component is made of stainless steel, with cement holding the two pegs. The upper tibial plateau is also cemented into position and is made of a high density plastic.

108. A-P radiograph of the tibia and fibula showing a giant cell tumour of the fibula.

109. A-P view of the knee showing osteochondritis dissecans involving medial femoral condyle. The femoral condyle seen on the left of the picture manifests a small area of increased bone density surrounded by an area of rarefaction.

110. A-P view of the knee showing fracture of the lateral tibial plateau held in good position by two lag screws and washers.

111. A-P view of knee joint indicating dislocation of the patella. Note the patella has been displaced laterally and is almost in line with the fibula.

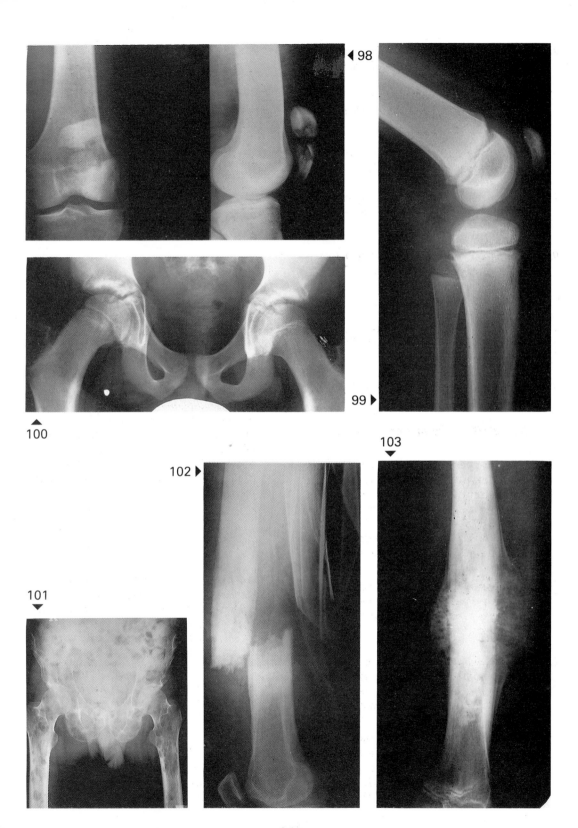

112. A-P view of upper tibia showing a large lytic metastasis that has arisen from carcinoma of the thyroid gland.

113. A-P radiograph of lower half of femur demonstrating chronic osteomyelitis. Note the thickening of the cortex and absence of a medullary cavity with irregularity of the lower femoral contour together with a lytic area in the lower central part of the femur.

114. A-P view of the lower femur showing osteochondroma growing away from the joint towards the pelvis in a late teenager. The lesion is seen on the right side of the picture in the mid section.

115. A-P view of a normal knee joint.

116. Lateral radiograph of knee joint showing gross osteoarthritis.

117. Diagrammatic representation of a semimembranosus bursa. Note it is tense in extension and softens on flexing the knee.

118. An oblique radiograph of the knee joint demonstrating osteochondritis dissecans.

119. Tear of the medial meniscus. One, the normal semi-lunar cartilage. Two, the bucket handled tear. Note the torn section is on the left hand side of the picture. Three, an anterior horn tear and Four, is a posterior horn tear.

120. Lateral view of tibia demonstrating a fracture at the junction of upper and lower halves with a butterfly fragment.

121. A-P radiograph of a tibia and fibula showing an oblique spiral fracture in the lower third of the tibia, and crack in upper tibia.

122. Lateral and A-P radiographs demonstrating a spiral fracture of the lower third of the tibia – seen more clearly in the A-P view on the right.

123. A-P view of a transverse fracture of the tibia held with plate and four screws. This fracture would have been better serviced with a plate and six screws that would have given greater stability.

124. A-P radiograph of ankle in which a fractured medial malleolus has been held in perfect position by means of a lag screw.

125. A-P view of an ankle demonstrating a Pott's fracture with involvement of the medial malleolus and lateral shift of the talus, and fractured fibula.

126. A-P and lateral aspects of normal metatarsal bones and phalanges.

127. A-P radiograph of foot showing hallux valgus with bunion formation and osteoarthritis of the metatarsophalangeal joint together with metatarsus primus varus. Metatarsus primus varus refers to the abnormally large gap or angulation between first and second metatarsals and the hallux valgus is indicated by the lateral angulation of the proximal phalanx in relation to the first metatarsal.

128. Lateral view of a normal calcaneum. Note Bohler's angle.

129. Lateral view showing fracture of the calcaneum. Note that Bohler's angle has been increased towards the direction of a straight angle or 180 degrees.

130. Lateral view of ankle region depicting fracture of neck of talus and avascular necrosis or death of the body of that bone. Note the dead body of talus directly below or inferior to the tibia and is shown to be densely white indicating avascular necrosis.

131. Diagrammatic representation indicating hammering of the second toe with callosity formation on the dorsal aspect of the skin overlying the proximal interphalangeal joint.

132. Lateral view of calcaneum showing fracture of body of calcaneum and flattening of Bohler's angle.

133. Diagrammatic representation of Monteggia fracture. Note the fracture is in the upper third of the ulna and is angled forward thus dislocating the head of the radius anteriorly out of its normal relationship with the elbow joint.

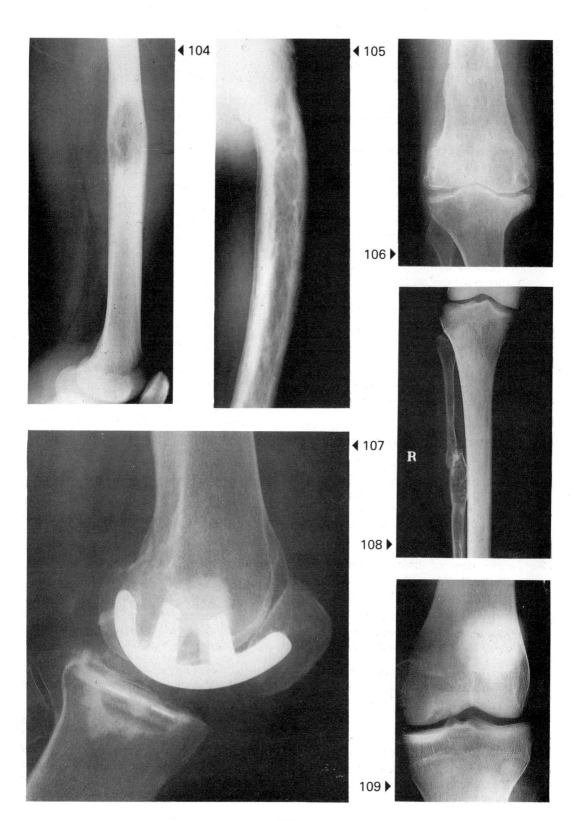

◀ 104

◀ 105

106 ▶

◀ 107

R

108 ▶

109 ▶

251

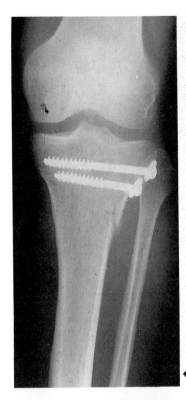

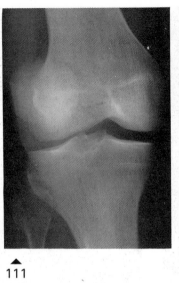

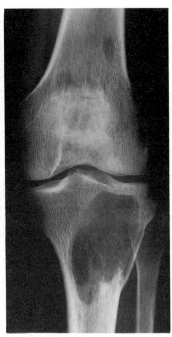

111

110

112

113

114 115

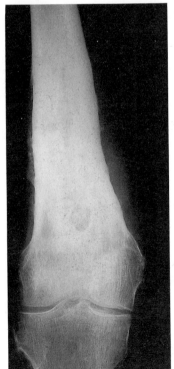

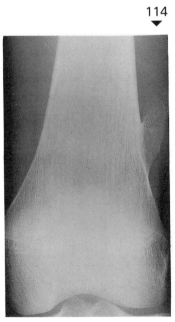

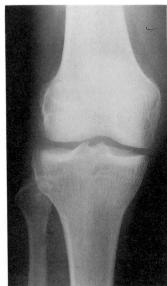

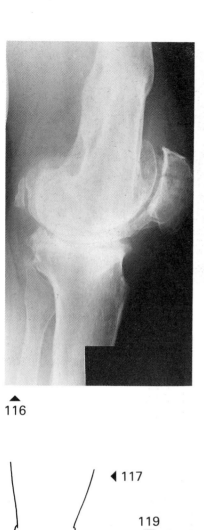

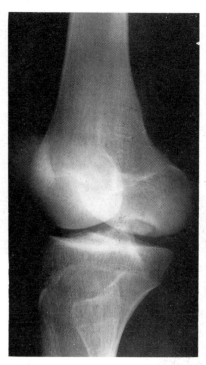

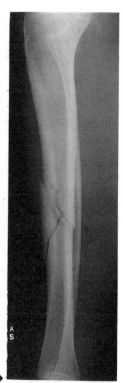

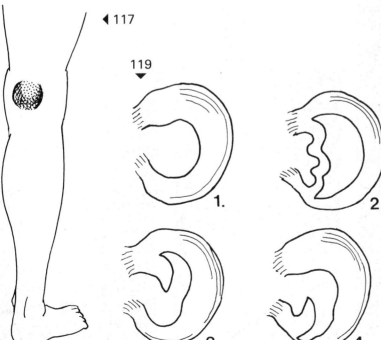

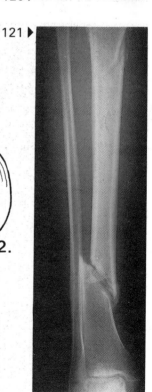

116

118

120 ▶

121 ▶

◀ 117

119
▼

1.

2.

3.

4.

253

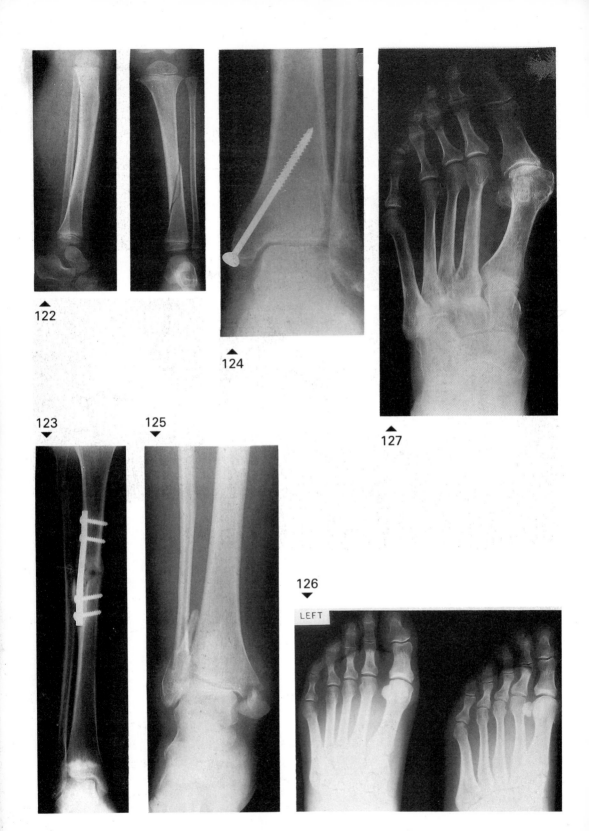

▲
122

▲
124

▲
127

123
▼

125
▼

126
▼

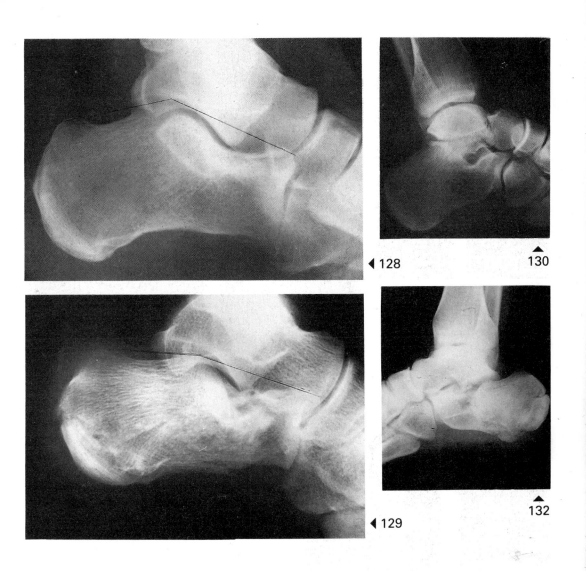

◀ 128

▲ 130

◀ 129

▲ 132

131
▼

133
▼

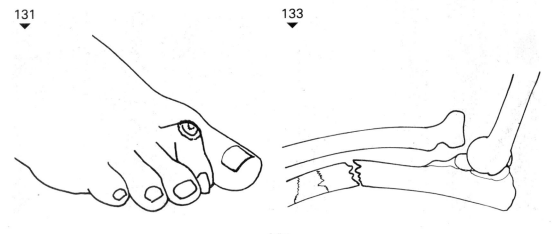